P9-DKF-991

The Complete Guide
to Stress Management

The Complete Guide to Stress Management

Dr. Chandra Patel

Plenum Press • New York and London

Library of Congress Cataloging-in-Publication Data

Patel, Chandra.
    The complete guide to stress management / Chandra Patel.
        p.   cm.
    Includes bibliographical references and index.
    ISBN 0-306-43967-0
    1. Stress management. 2. Stress (Psychology)   I. Title.
RA785.P38   1991
 155.9'042--dc20   91-20027
                                                            CIP

ISBN 0-306-43967-0

© 1991 Chandra Patel
Plenum Press is a division of Plenum Publishing Corporation
233 Spring Street, New York, N.Y. 10013

All rights reserved

No part of this book may be reproduced, stored in a retrieval system, or transmitted
in any form or by any means, electronic, mechanical, photocopying, microfilming,
recording, or otherwise, without written permission from the Publisher

Printed in the United States of America

Dedicated to
Param Pujya Pramukhswami Maharaj

Foreword

The field of stress illustrates, better than most, some of the tensions that pervade the growing public interest in health. We have witnessed some extreme positions: intense public interest in stress and a thirst for information, contrasted with doctors' unwillingness to do more than prescribe tranquilizers; "scientists" who make a career of trendy newsworthy studies of burnout and whole occupations crippled by stress, set against a professional reluctance to recognize that there is a scientific field of endeavor here and hence any ground for a professional opinion; practitioners who are confronted by everyday experiences of stress, compared with careful academics for whom all the evidence is not yet in; champions of alternative therapy who see it as part of a critique of allopathic medicine, Western Science, and perhaps a good part of Western civilization as well, ranged against keepers of the faith of orthodox medicine.

Perhaps these tensions and entrenched positions are a necessary part of the growth of knowledge and the working out of the strengths and limitations of various approaches to health problems. They may be good for the growth of knowledge for the committed to defend their positions with religious fervor, but they may not be so good for people who now want help in finding their way through the maze of media hype and conflicting views.

Chandra Patel has remarkable qualifications for providing such a guide. She bridges many of the divides listed above. She is not only a practitioner who developed her ideas through experience of everyday treatment of patients with problems, but also an academic trained in the methods of scientific investigation. She is a doctor trained and skilled in the practice of Western medicine who has not lost her insights gained from an Eastern view of the world. She is a developer of new holistic approaches to care who has subjected them to that archetypical symbol of scientific medicine: the randomized controlled trial.

Her scientific investigations into nonpharmacological control of hypertension may be one of the better examples of keeping the baby while discarding the bathwater. They illustrate why she may have special insight into the problems of stress that may be of practical use to people. As a general practitioner, she felt that people with hypertension needed some treatment resource other than permanent recourse to drugs. She therefore developed her Yoga-based relaxation technique. Over time this developed in two ways. It became more than simply a technique for relaxation; it became a stress-management package, designed to recognize the sources of stress and, where possible, to deal with them, in addition to counteracting their bodily effects. The second development was increasingly rigorous scientific evaluation of the technique. It was demonstrated that it could be taught in groups at work, as well as to individual patients in general practice, and that other therapists could be trained to teach the technique, with a consequent benefit to people with mild hypertension: keeping them off drugs without a rise in blood pressure.

This book attempts to bring the knowledge gained from twenty years of investigation and treatment to a wider audience. Chandra Patel's combination of wise insight, scientific knowledge, and wide practical experience makes her especially qualified to write it. It is likely to provide help to a wide range of people.

Michael Marmot

University College, London

Acknowledgments

This book gives a detailed account of the advice I have given to individuals who have consulted me as a medical practitioner over the last twenty years, and of the behavior modification programs I have run for patients believed to have high blood pressure or an increased risk of having a heart attack in the future, or for those who have already suffered heart attacks or other cardiovascular complications. I have also offered this program to those suffering from other stress-related conditions, like migraine and tension headaches, as well as discomfort associated with anxiety states related to coping with exceptionally difficult situations in life. Many have participated in research trials. Their enthusiastic cooperation and willingness to allow themselves to be experimented on have been instrumental in shaping my beliefs, clarifying many thoughts and concepts, and providing me with the creative energy necessary to conduct many scientific studies as well as to work as a clinician. I am deeply indebted to them. The scientific studies could not have been carried out without the kind help and support of my numerous colleagues, and I sincerely thank them.

Over the years, I have been inspired and nurtured by the work of numerous investigators and authors, only a few of whom are referred to in the book and listed in the bibliography. I particularly wish to thank the following authors, for their work which I have greatly plundered. Robert Bramson for *Coping with Difficult People;* Lewis Smedes for *Forget and Forgive;* Holly Atkinson for *Women and Fatigue;* Gwain Shakti for *Creative Visualisation;* James House for *Work Stress and Social Support;* Lawrence LeShan for *How to Meditate;* Matthew McKay and Patrick Fanning for *Self-Esteem;* Swami Rama, Rudolph Ballentine, and Alan Hymes for *Science of Breath;* and Meyer Friedman and Ray Rosenman for *Type A Behavior and Your Heart.*

I also wish to thank Erica Smith for reading the first draft and making useful suggestions, and, last but not the least, I would like to thank my husband, Hiru, who has patiently endured me, willingly taken a bigger share in family commitments, and actively supported me through my extraordinarily demanding career and research pursuits.

Contents

Part II. How to Cope with Stress

Introduction

An old man once called his two sons and told them, "Sons, I am getting old now and I must decide to which one of you I should entrust my business and properties when I am gone. So I am going to set you a little test. To each of you, I give five coins. There are two empty storerooms at the back of our garden. With the money I give you, I want each of you to fill up a room by the time I come back tomorrow morning."

The older son thought, "The old man is getting senile. What can you get for five coins that can fill up an entire room? Rubbish?" And as he was talking to himself, a thought flashed through his mind. He went to see some trash collectors and told them, "I want you to bring all the rubbish from the village tonight and fill up my storeroom, and I will give you five coins." The trash collectors thought he was crazy, but they had nothing to lose. In fact, they could save some time by not having to take the rubbish all the way to the rubbish dump, and they would get five coins as well! So they agreed.

The next day the father came back to see what his sons had done with the money he had given them. He went first to the older son, who told his father that he would be very pleased with what he had done, for he had managed to fill the entire room. Upon smelling the stench, the father quickly closed the door and went to see the younger son.

The younger son had bought a candle, some incense sticks, and a flute, and he was sitting in a candlelit room with burning incense, playing the flute. He had filled the room with light, fragrance, and sweet music. I am sure you have guessed to which of the sons the father left his business. The point I wish to make, however, is that each one of us has been given the priceless gift of life, and it is up to us what we fill that life with. Will it be aggravations, disappointment, despair, and dissatisfaction or will it be joy, peace, happiness, and love? If you wish it to be the latter, you will find this book helpful.

This book aims to help the reader understand what stress is, how it is caused, how to recognize stress symptoms, and, finally, how to reduce its impact on health and well-being by using learned strategies. Although "stress" is difficult to define precisely and even more difficult to measure, we know enough about it to be able to do something positive to alleviate it. Stress is caused not only by external factors, which are called *stressors*, but is also generated internally by our hopes and aspirations, beliefs and attitudes, as well as by our personality attributes and by our unrealistic expectations of ourselves. Stress occurs at work, at home, and in our social life. Even though we like to think that we live autonomous lives, we are affected by a wide variety of national and international economic, political, and ecological factors. Although we may have little control over our environment, how we respond to our environment, or how we allow it to affect us, is entirely our own responsibility.

In order to reduce stress, we need first to be aware of the factors which cause stress in our life and how they may strain our health. Whenever possible, we need to remove stressors, or at least to reduce their quantity or severity. We need to make our environment more tolerable, safe, and balanced to bring about political, economic, and social changes, and to reduce our vulnerability and increase our resistance to stress. Removing stressors may not be easy, but if we are aware of them, we can certainly try to avoid those that are unnecessary or, if that is not possible or even desirable, at least to anticipate them and plan ahead for the best possible way of confronting them.

Changing an uncomfortable or unsafe physical environment may be very difficult and may require considerable skill in communication and assertiveness to secure the cooperation of employers, unions, or other agencies. It is also important that we balance work with leisure activities. For example, if our work is strenuous, involving standing, walking, lifting, or bending all day long, we need a nonphysical leisure time activity. If, on the other hand, our work requires us to sit at a desk all day, a leisure time activity involving exercise is the best way to balance our environment.

Equally, it may not be easy to arrange a congenial psychological environment. If our job is unrewarding or unfulfilling, we can try to make it more interesting by our own efforts, by enlisting the cooperation of others, or by developing a philosophical or positive mental attitude toward it. Learning to talk things over with people we trust or with specialized counselors can do amazing things for a shaky marriage or other social and personal problems.

Interpersonal conflicts cause a considerable amount of stress. Who are these people who create stress in our lives? Possible descriptions, as well as some suggestions for ways of coping with those difficult people who create havoc in our lives, are given in the last chapter. It is unlikely that we can change the political, social, or economic climate of the country single-handed, but awareness and understanding of how they affect our lives can ease the confusion. Increased public awareness is necessary before changes can be expected or pressures exerted to bring about change. A detailed discussion of such forces is beyond the scope of this book.

The best possible strategies for reducing stress are those we can undertake ourselves. How can we increase our resistance to stress? Here again, it is important to be aware of factors which increase our susceptibility so that we can avoid them or at least anticipate them. We can go even further. A variety of physical and mental relaxation techniques are available which can be easily learned. They directly counteract the effect of stress. Similarly, altering stressful behavior or complex emotions like anger and hostility can counteract factors which make us vulnerable.

However, such behavior modification or reduction of tension through relaxation is only the tip of the iceberg. Hidden below the tip lies the mass of our problem: our beliefs, our attitudes, our expectations of ourselves and others, and the deep motivation that drives us to do things in a certain less-than-ideal way. It is these that we need to tackle to bring about lasting relief from stress, and to exploit more fully our enormous human potential.

If it is difficult to define and measure stress, it is even more difficult to calculate its cost. It costs an inordinate amount in terms of human misery. Eight out of every ten persons surveyed in a recent national poll said that they need less stress in their lives. Several hundred studies have shown a relationship between stress, such as divorce or change in career, and development of disease. In addition to absenteeism, stress leads to poor industrial relations, poor productivity, conflicts, official and unofficial strikes, high staff turnover, job dissatisfaction, and industrial accidents. A government report recommended that at least 30 percent of the 500 largest companies in the United States should offer a stress management program by 1990.

Many of the strategies described in this book have been tried and tested by me and my colleagues in scientific studies. If you can motivate yourself to follow the strategies given in this book and continue with them, our research suggests that you are likely to achieve some of the following.

- Reduced level of anxiety
- Reduction in the level of blood pressure
- Reduction in the intensity and frequency of headaches

- Better quality of sleep
- Reduction in the risk of having heart attacks
- Better relationships with people at work
- Improved general health
- Greater enjoyment of life
- Better personal and family relationships
- Improvement in the level of physical energy
- Better sexual life
- Improved concentration at work
- Improvement in mental well-being
- Better social life

This book is primarily addressed directly to the public. It is based on my personal experience as a health care provider who has successfully validated the stress management program described in this book in randomized controlled trials. Therefore, a variety of health care workers—psychologists, counselors, physicians, nurses, social workers, occupational therapists, physiotherapists, and others involved in helping patients to alleviate stress—would find this book useful.

Furthermore, senior-level management, work supervisors, line managers, shop stewards, and union bosses will become more aware of the sources and frequency of stress at work and its impact on the health and morale of employees. However, more than that, they will better understand the crucial roles they can play in stress management at work, not only in terms of established channels of authority and communication, but also by training themselves or other key personnel to serve as sources of social support and providers of stress management skills.

Note: Throughout this book the masculine pronoun *he* is used when referring to the doctor or the patient. This is merely for convenience and includes *she* as well.

Numbers in brackets appearing in the text refer to entries in the Bibliography.

I

Causes and Consequences of Stress

1

What Is Stress?

People everywhere have long been interested in a wide range of phenomena called *stress*. It is a concept which is familiar to both laypeople and the medical profession, but although most people understand its meaning in general terms, it is very difficult to define precisely. No single definition has been fully able to capture the nature of this complex concept. However, stress not only can be imposed by external demands but can also be generated from within by our hopes, fears, expectations, and beliefs. It follows that what is stressful to one person may be a refreshing challenge to another, depending upon his perception of the situation as well as his perception of his ability to cope with that situation.

The individual's judgment that a stressful situation exists, whether or not it appears so to an outsider, is important in initiating a stress response (23). Without this appraisal there is no stress in the person's psychological schema. Even though a situation is perceived as a demand or threat it may still not mobilize a stress response if the individual thinks that he is able to cope with it adequately, either on his own or with the help of external resources or support from other people in his life. In general, the balance resulting from the interaction of these four components—external demands, internal needs and values, personal coping resources, and external resources or support—determines whether a particular situation will be stressful or not.

Once a situation has been assessed as demanding or frustrating, it will engender a comprehensive physiological response which has mental, emotional, physical, and behavioral components. The intensity of this stress response varies, and we may not always be consciously aware of it. The final outcome of the stress response may have implications when similar pressures are encountered in the future (see diagram on page 11).

"Stress," then, is a specific response the body makes to all nonspecific demands. Instances include important challenges (e.g., making an important presentation), being exposed to threat (e.g., when our competence is questioned), or struggling to meet unrealistic expectations of others as well as our own (e.g., we are expected to be a competent manager when, in fact, we are superb at our craft but not good at managing, or we strive to be perfect in all things). No matter what the situation is, when the demand we perceive exceeds the resources we think we have, the body and mind are aroused and all systems are geared up either to fight the challenge (often successfully) or to flee from the situation to avoid harm. A certain amount of stress occurs all the time. There is no life without stress. However, when people complain about stress, they are talking of too much stress or of having symptoms of stress.

NOT ALL STRESS IS BAD FOR US

Some stress is essential for our very existence as well as for our continued personal growth. A completely unstressed person might as well be dead. A certain amount of stress gives us a zest for life and releases our creativity. Having too few challenges makes our lives boring and frustrating: this can be

MODEL OF HUMAN STRESS

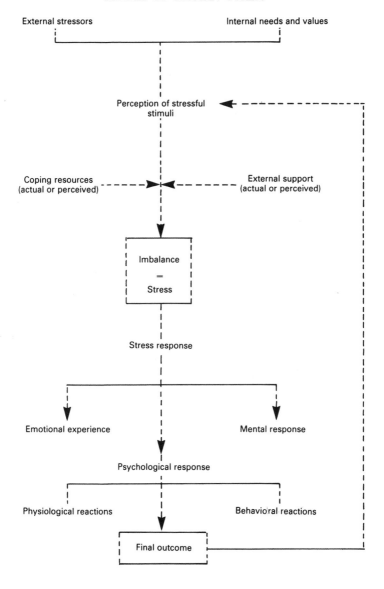

THE HUMAN PERFORMANCE CURVE

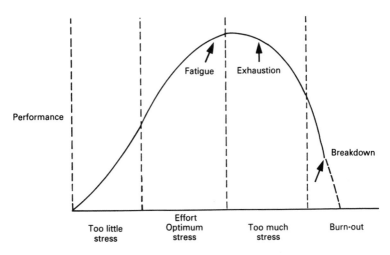

unproductive and just as stressful as having too many challenges. It has been said that finding the right balance is like adjusting the strings of a musical instrument: too loose and the tune will be ruined, too tight and the strings will break.

Any situation which the individual perceives to be psychologically or physically demanding involves active coping. Successful coping will improve performance up to a certain point, after which there is no further improvement, but neither is there any deterioration, as coping efforts are matched to the person's tolerance level. However, if changes come too fast to allow adequate time for the person to adapt, he may begin to experience warning signs suggesting that he is overstretched or overburdened. If he continues his efforts and his initial symptoms of fatigue or other stress indicators are ignored, he may reach a point where a breakdown in health or a "burn-out" syndrome is likely to occur. This normal human reaction to stress is shown in the diagram above.

The Human Performance Curve

Too Little Stress. In this situation there is insufficient challenge to achieve a sense of personal accomplishment. Skills are underutilized. Lack of stimulation leads to boredom. There is a lack of purpose or meaning in life.

Optimum Stress. Life is balanced and, despite ups and downs, perfectly manageable. Job satisfaction and a sense of achievement enable the person to cruise through daily work without much difficulty and to be pleasantly tired at the end of the day.

Too Much Stress. There is a constant feeling of having too much to do every day. Despite emotional and physical exhaustion the person is unable to take time off to rest and play. He is in permanent overdrive but not achieving results as expected.

Breakdown. If his efforts are continued the person may develop chronic neurotic tendencies or one of several psychosomatic illnesses. Excessive stress may show up in excessive drinking or smoking, or in reliance on tranquilizers or sleeping pills. Accidents may occur at work or at home as the stressed individual is likely to be preoccupied with unresolved tensions. He may attack others or incite others to attack him. Sometimes opposite reactions may occur. As relationships deteriorate, the person may become withdrawn. If these signs are recognized by the individual or by those who surround him and appropriate steps are taken, he may pull himself out of disequilibrium, and mental or physical tragedies will be avoided. If, on the other hand, he continues his efforts despite exhaustion, he is likely to have a mental or physical breakdown. Severe depression and coronary heart attack are examples of such breakdowns.

Keeping the Balance

Hans Selye, often known as the father of stress research, described these four stages, respectively, as understress, eustress, overstress, and distress (121), and suggested that we need to recognize our own eustress, when our bodies and minds are in balance, and when we feel energetic, adaptable, approachable, and relaxed. When we cross the boundary, we are likely to feel tired, anxious, aggressive, or defensive. We need a balance. Life is not a short hundred-yard dash, requiring a short spurt of intense effort to win. Life is a marathon: the more care you take over how you use your energy by making necessary adjustments, the less you waste it and the longer your reserves will last. Remember, you have only one life.

Stress Can Be Positive or Negative

Anything that is new evokes a stress response as the body and mind prepare to meet the unknown challenge. However, some events are associated with positive emotions while others engender negative emotions. Examples of positive emotions are pleasure, enthusiasm, mastery, excitement, confidence, happiness, joy, love, and intellectual stimulation; negative emotions include fear, anxiety, hate, resentment, conflict, uncertainty, irritation, jealousy, frustration, guilt, rage, fury, boredom, and dissatisfaction. Even joy and excitement mobilize the same adrenaline response as negative emotions but on the whole the threshold is much higher (i.e., more joy and excitement are needed to produce the same adrenaline response). Positive feelings like pleasure and mastery can actually improve our resistance to stress, while negative feelings like uncertainty or dissatisfaction lower it.

If we are happy or confident, if we take time to appreciate the pleasures offered by life and by the people around us, we have lots of energy. Even though the things that happen to us can be unpredictable and may be both positive and negative, we can increase our threshold for stress symptoms like pain or fatigue by planning activities which maximize our pleasure in life. Music, relaxation, pleasant conversation with a friend, adequate sleep, having a picnic, an evening of dancing, and going to a museum can increase our resistance to stress. Similarly, a sense of humor increases our capacity to withstand challenges and adversities.

Examples of Positive Stress

- Feeling confident we will overcome a challenge
- Feeling exhilarated and invigorated by a competitive sport
- Getting a promotion we have been waiting for
- Winning a football pool
- Being involved in a new love affair

Examples of Negative Stress

- Having to learn a difficult task
- Being stuck in a traffic jam
- Having a secretary be out sick
- Having a child with measles
- Having a computer break down

WHO EXPERIENCES STRESS?

All of us encounter challenge, threat, or annoyance in the course of daily life. Occasionally these can be life-threatening, but more often they simply threaten our pride, our prestige, our position at work, our place in the family or society, and our self-image. Even though the popular image of an over-worked or overstressed person is of a highly placed executive, research has shown that people who suffer from stress are scattered among all social classes and are of both sexes and all ages. From that point of view a burned-out executive does not differ from a depressed, apathetic, prematurely aged un-employed person or assembly-line worker. It is the following aspects that vary across people.

The Way Each Individual Perceives the Situation

Genetic background, past experience, family upbringing, and cultural background, as well as present circumstances, all influence the way a situation is evaluated and thus responded to. We may call this the psychobiological programming of the person. What feels like an overwhelming situation to one per-son may be a stimulating challenge to another and a mere trifle to a third.

How an Individual Copes with a Given Situation

Our individual training and our expectations of ourselves or others contribute to the way we cope. One person may be inclined to conform to the demands of society, another may rebel against all rules and regulations, and another may try to reform society—if necessary, single-handedly.

The Actual Situation Which Causes Stress

An administrator may be affected by quite different events from a worker. However, it is not the situation itself but its meaning that is important. External stressors, together with psychobiological programming, determine the occur-rence of the stress response, which may lead to precursors of disease and then disease itself unless appropriate action is taken.

How the Individual Experiences Stress—Physically, Mentally, Emotionally, or Behaviorally

People differ both in the intensity with which they react to environmental factors and in the pattern of their reaction.

WHERE AND WHEN DOES STRESS OCCUR?

Occasionally, a crisis occurs in life when stress is understandable and inevitable. Examples include bereavement or being fired after twenty years of work. However, most stress is not related to life crises. Predominantly, the energy we expend on trivia or relentless daily annoyances cumulatively make a major impact on our health and functioning. The following are examples:

- Getting up late because the alarm failed to go off
- Coping with a hot-water tank that starts leaking
- Being repeatedly interrupted by telephone calls when we are trying to meet an important deadline
- Noisy roadwork when our job requires total concentration
- The car's not starting when we are late for work
- Being stuck in a traffic jam
- Being involved in a minor accident but having to spend hours making a report to the police
- Having a demanding time schedule

UNDERSTANDING STRESS PHYSIOLOGY

Animals, when confronted with an overwhelming stress or alarming situation, such as the sudden appearance of a predator, respond in a split second. They usually respond in one of two ways, depending on their perception of the situation. If they perceive their own strength to be sufficient to make victory a distinct possibility, they get ready to fight the predator. If, on the other hand, they feel that the battle is likely to be lost they prepare to flee. This alarm response is also known as the *fight-or-flight response*. A third response, freezing, may occasionally occur: the animal sits still as if paralyzed by fear.

Human beings are not much different. Whether the threat is physical, mental, or emotional, the body responds by preparing itself for fight or flight. The sense organs of sight and hearing receive signals from external situations and pass them on to a specific area of the brain surface known as the *sensory cortex*. The information received by the sensory cortex is integrated with other data stored in memory files and is evaluated. If the final evaluation is of demand, challenge, or threat, the primitive brain (known as the *hypothalamus*) is activated. Nerve impulses from the hypothalamus go to the adrenal medulla—the core of the adrenal glands, which are situated above the kidneys—as well as directly to every muscle, blood vessel, and organ in the body. In response to this stimulation the adrenal medulla secretes stress hormones called epinephrine and norepinephrine, which are collectively known as *catecholamines*. The hypothalamus also produces a chemical called *corticotropin-releasing factor* (CRF), which stimulates the pituitary gland at the base of the brain to produce adrenocorticotropic hormone (ACTH). This activates the adrenal cortex (the outer part of the adrenal gland), which in turn releases another hormone, known as *cortisol*. These hormones circulate through the bloodstream and reach every organ and activate every cell in the body to gear them up for action (see the flowchart on page 21). The changes occurring in the body may themselves affect our perception and hence how we continue to respond to persisting demands.

Primitive Stress Response

The protective mechanism which immediately springs into operation when our life is threatened is built in. It prepares us for a fight-or-flight response and involves the following biological changes:

- The liver releases sugar and fats which flow into the bloodstream to provide fuel for quick energy.
- Respiration becomes faster, so more oxygen is provided.
- Red blood cells flood the bloodstream, carrying more oxygen to the muscles of the limbs and the brain.
- The heart beats faster and the blood pressure rises, so that sufficient blood reaches the necessary areas. This response can sometimes be felt as a pounding heart or a racing pulse. If the threat is overwhelming, the heart may, paradoxically, slow down and, in a critical condition, may even stop.
- Blood-clotting mechanisms are activated in anticipation of injury. Nature provided this mechanism to protect us in the Stone Age, when we were more likely to be fighting a saber-toothed tiger and, without this clotting mechanism, would have bled to death. The mechanism ensures that clots will seal up the injured blood vessels. Nowadays, an increased clotting tendency may well cause thrombosis in blood vessels and lead to a heart attack or a stroke.
- The muscles become tense in preparation for strenuous action. For example, the shoulder may be braced, the muscles are tense in readiness to run, the body may become rigid, and the fists and jaw are clenched ready to fight.
- Saliva dries up and digestion ceases, so that blood may be diverted to the muscles and brain, where it is needed

most. The stomach may become flabby and give a sinking feeling. Gastric juice secretion may increase and may be felt as a burning sensation in the pit of the stomach.

- Perspiration increases so that the body may cool down. This makes sense when we consider that fighting makes us feel very hot and that, without a cooling mechanism, our body temperature would rise steeply.
- The bowel and bladder muscles may become loose.
- The pupils dilate, so that more light enters and we can see in the dark.
- All senses are heightened, so that we can make swift decisions and take action.

The person who undergoes these changes is in a prime state of readiness to deal with danger, challenge, or other real or imaginary demands. However, this state is a temporary one, reserved for extreme situations, and the body cannot maintain it as a lasting condition. Once the immediate threat is removed or overcome, or after we have adapted to the disturbance, a reverse mechanism is activated and the body returns to its normal state. If the stressor persists, or if resistance continues after the stressor is removed, the alarm stage can be prolonged, and health may be temporarily or even permanently damaged.

Laboratory experiments have shown that similar changes occur in human beings in a variety of stressful situations. For example, catecholamine secretions are increased by noise, electric shock, parachute jumping, traveling in crowded trains, performing tasks under time pressure, and situations of conflict. It is not the physical characteristics of the situation that are important but its emotional impact on the individual. For example, the same adrenomedullary response is mobilized whether the stress is due to too much work or to the boredom of too little work. Both situations produce similar results because they are both disturbing experiences. Epinephrine is more sensitive to mental stress while norepinephrine is more sensitive to physical stress like exercise or exposure to cold.

STRESS RESPONSE PATHWAY

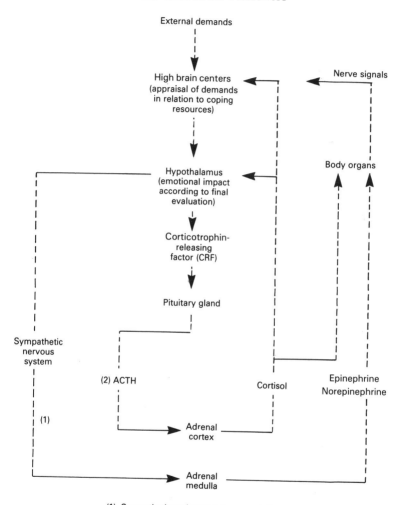

(1) Sympathetic pathway: adrenomedullary system
(2) Pituitary pathway: adrenocortical system

It is also important to remember that epinephrine goes up not just during anger or fear but also to some extent during elation and amusement.

The pituitary-adrenal-cortical system is stimulated in human beings when they are exposed to novel and unfamiliar situations which evoke feelings of uncertainty, helplessness, and anxiety, while predictability or controllability of the events can suppress the secretion of cortisol. Anticipation is a powerful stimulus for cortisol release as it involves a certain amount of uncertainty. In a study by Marianne Frankenhaeuser (35) of children taking psychological tests, half of the children were told that during the test they would be briefly separated from their parents. The anxiety induced by this threat was reflected in their having a significantly higher level of cortisol despite the fact that they never were actually separated.

Recently, it has been recognized that stress can also affect the body's immune system, which protects us from invasion by foreign substances called *antigens* by making protective substances called *antibodies*. In addition, fighter cells, known as *natural killer cells*, seek out and destroy cells that have acquired foreign characteristics, such as infected or cancer cells. Researchers have found an impairment in natural-killer-cell activity in bereaved women (5). Potentially damaging changes have also been found in the helper cells known as *T-lymphocytes*, which, as the word *helper* implies, also play an important role in defending against antigens.

This stress response is also associated with mental, emotional, and behavioral changes. Mental changes vary from increased alertness and ability to make swift decisions to memory lapses and rash judgment. Emotional changes can include irritation, anger, fear, hostility, and even rage and fury. Behaviorally, the person may become aggressive.

There are two major components of stress experience: effort and distress (35). The effort factor involves elements of interest, engagement, and determination. It implies active coping, that is, striving to gain and maintain control. The distress factor involves elements of dissatisfaction, boredom, uncertainty, and anxiety. It is associated with a passive attitude and a feeling of helplessness. Effort is associated with an increase in catecholamine, while distress is mainly associated with a rise in cortisol, which is much more damaging. Effort and distress can be experienced together or they may be experienced one at a time.

Effort with distress is associated with an increase in both catecholamine and cortisol. This is a typical state when we are striving to gain and maintain control over daily hassles or irritations. In working life it commonly occurs in people engaged in repetitive, machine-paced jobs on an assembly line or in a highly routine, monotonous job like working at a computer terminal. Effort without distress is a joyous state; there is a high degree of job involvement; active, successful coping; and a sense of having adequate personal control. It is accompanied by release of catecholamine, but cortisol secretion is suppressed. Distress without effort implies helplessness, loss of control, or giving up. In this state cortisol secretion is high while catecholamine may be high or low. This is a typical profile of a depressed patient.

Complexities of the Human Brain

The primitive stress response described above is common to all mammals. It has been observed in animals and confirmed in laboratory experiments. In civilized man, however, the dangers are rarely life-threatening, and the primitive response is often inappropriate. Modern humans possess the complex dimension of the mind which has the ability to interpret a situation through an array of beliefs, attitudes, and expectations. This ability provides an infinite variety of ways to react to stressors. Thus, threats not only to life but also to our pride and our position in society or in the family result in psychological and subjective experiences (like frustration, conflict, fear, or anger) and their accompanying behavioral components (like arguments, aggression, sarcastic remarks, or withdrawal), which combine with the physiological or biological components of the stress response. The degree of this response depends on the threatening value we put on the situation and our ability to adapt.

Adaptation: Success or Failure

Most life changes evoke this stress response, which prepares an individual for active coping. This is the basis of learning through experience. When a situation recurs repeatedly the brain consciously or subconsciously interprets the repeated stimuli as either irrelevant or relevant. In the latter case, the individual will bring an active coping response into play, and thus the stimulus will lose its threatening value. Through repeated stimuli and readjustments equilibrium is maintained most of the time. The process of adaptation is, however, more complex and varies considerably from person to person. Earlier positive or negative experiences may help or hinder the process of adaptation.

For example, Dr. Martin Seligman (120) showed in laboratory experiments that previous exposure to an unsolvable situation in which all the appropriate responses have been futile leads to the belief that coping or trying to cope is irrelevant to the outcome and hence there is no point in trying to respond. This failure to adapt often manifests itself in the characteristics of helplessness and apathy and is the basis of the saying "once bitten, twice shy." Occasionally, previous failure may lead to greater effort on further exposure. If demands are continuous the body and mind may become overwhelmed with the number of changes having to be made. In that state, it may take only a minor incident to push us over the edge. If such adaptive responses are prolonged, intense, or frequently repeated, they increase wear and tear, exhaust the body of its adaptive energy, and may eventually damage the structure and function of one or more organs in the body. The final effect may be serious illness of the body or the mind or even death.

Stress and the Individual

Everyone's perception of what constitutes a threat or demand is different. It is not only actual coping ability but also the perception of one's ability to cope that is important. These perceptions have a lot to do with how much or how well or badly we react to a situation. We all have a different tolerance level. What one person finds extremely stressful and succumbs to, another may find tolerable, and yet another may positively thrive on. For our own health, it is our duty to consider whether our reactions are likely to be beneficial or harmful, dangerous to ourselves or others, and what the outcome will be, in the short or long run. If a harmful outcome is predicted we should take appropriate steps and do all within our power to prevent damage.

2

Stressors
The Factors That Cause Stress

Stressors are the factors in our lives which induce the stress response. We commonly use the term *stress* to mean both stressors and the stress response. Stressors occur at work, at home, or in our social life and are sometimes referred to as *external environments*.

LIFE EVENTS AND WHAT THEY MEAN

Any new event in life generally causes stress, as the individual tries to adjust to the demands made by those events. Adaptation involves the use of resources and the depletion of energy. As our reserves are depleted our resistance to disease is lowered and our susceptibility to illness increases. Some events are more stressful than others, depending on the degree of adaptation required. When changes happen in rapid succession, they increase an individual's vulnerability. Research by Harold G. Wolff (144) indicated that stressful life events are important in causing illness by evoking biological reactions and that this link applies not only to psychosomatic disorders but also to more organic pathology like infections, as well as accidents and injuries. Further studies by Meyer and Haggarty (90) showed, for example, that respiratory illnesses were four times as likely to be preceded as followed by acute stress. Then, Drs. Thomas Holmes and Richard Rahe (57) developed a method of tabulating and quantifying life changes, which they tested on over 5,000 patients.

Holmes and Rahe observed that life's events tend to cluster or increase in intensity prior to the onset of disease. The greater the amount of social readjustment, the greater the likelihood of developing an illness, not only severe illness but also minor complaints like cuts and bruises, headaches, backaches, colds, and coughs. In one study of 2,500 officers and enlisted men aboard three naval cruisers, Dr. Rahe (109) found that the 30 percent of the men with the highest life-change scores developed 90 percent more illness during the first month of cruising than the 30 percent of men with the lowest life-change scores. In another study of eighty-four junior hospital doctors in the United States scores for life changes in the previous eighteen months were collected. Eight months later enquiries were made about their illnesses during the intervening months. The results showed that in the group with high life-change scores, 49 percent had experienced some illness; in the medium-score group, the figure was 25 percent; and in the low-score group, only 9 percent had been ill (56).

Some events deserve special mention. Disturbance in certain aspects of the immune function has been reported after bereavement, sleep deprivation, preexamination stress, and job loss, while other events boost immunity (141).

Bereavement

When someone we dearly love dies, especially if this happens suddenly, without any warning, our life instantly becomes a swirling chaos. "It felt as if a massive stone was placed on my chest," said Peggy when her husband died in a plane crash (30). "I was dazed and gripping to all those who were trying to make sense of what was happening to me." She couldn't stand being touched, tended to forget her friends' names, and had screaming nightmares. Sometimes she just wanted to die. Occasionally she felt she couldn't move her legs out of bed. Even weeks later, she was still devastated: "I was desperate to believe that my husband still existed, in some form, somewhere." Three months later, she still could not see an end to her desolation and was avoiding social meetings: "I was still having trouble concentrating and still declining invitations because I didn't have the energy to be witty and conversational." Grief, while not an illness, is a major threat to mental and physical health.

There is a common pattern to grief consisting of three stages: numbing, despair, and detachment. At first it is hard to believe that the loss has really happened; there may be a feeling of unreality about the things around us, including one's body. Sometimes the body may feel distanced and lifeless or not there at all. All feelings are numbed. Numbing lasts from a few hours to a few days. This is followed by despair, during which there are waves of strong feelings; every hour or so one feels intense sadness, intense anger, or intense love. Some cultures allow open grieving, which can release sorrow or rage, but when expression is denied, heavy pains may be felt in the chest or stomach, or in the entire body. There may be a feeling of tightness in the throat or a choking sensation. We may feel guilty and recriminate ourselves: "If only I had told him I loved him"; "If only I had called the doctor earlier, she would still be alive." Sometimes we imagine that we hear or see the dead person. We may even experience his last symptoms, and it is hard to be interested in anything. We may feel so restless that we pace up and down, wring our hands aimlessly, or sigh. We are constantly preoccupied with the past. Finally, there comes a point when we gradually begin to detach ourselves from the old ties. This is not to say that we forget the person; it is not a cold detachment but one which enables us to say good-bye to the person we once loved. We begin to take an interest in new things and adjust to the environment which is so different without our old friend or partner.

Life Events and Cardiovascular Incidents

Death from a broken heart may be a figure of speech from a bygone age, but Colin Murray Parkes and his colleagues (98) followed 4,486 widowers in Wales and found that grief could kill through the heart. The results showed that the death rate in these widowers was significantly higher in the first year of bereavement than in other men of the same ages. Most of these deaths were from heart attacks. Another study, by Cottington and co-workers (22) in Baltimore, showed that the recent death of someone significant in their lives was six times more common in women dying a sudden cardiac death than in healthy women of the same age. A similar study of women who had suffered heart attacks in Göteborg, Sweden, also showed that these women tended to have experienced more life events in the years preceding their heart attacks than healthy women of the same age. There have been many reports of people dying suddenly in conditions of overwhelming stress (32). The causes have been not only bereavement but also disaster, working during the day and going to college at night, getting divorced, going reluctantly to the dentist, and so on. In other words, these situations arouse overwhelming emotions that invoke an intense sense of threat, danger, loss, and, paradoxically, relief. The important factors in these situations are that they are unpredictable and that the individual has, or feels he has, no control over them.

When a number of survivors of heart attack were interviewed within three days of its onset, significantly more patients reported that they had experienced disturbing life events in the weeks prior to the heart attack than healthy subjects of similar ages. A group of Swedish researchers (135) followed up 6,723 building-construction workers and found that clusters of life events, like "workload" during the previous twelve months—which included conflicts and responsibility at work, extra work, and threat of unemployment—recent change in family structure, and chronic family difficulties were important predictors of heart attack. Workload also showed a connection with neurosis and low back pain (136).

Dr. Paykel (105) in England has shown that loss events, such as bereavement or the loss of a job, are more likely to be associated with illness than gain events, such as having a new family member. He, as well as other Swedish workers (74), have shown that it is not the amount of adjustment we have to make that is important but the amount of upset caused by a particular event. Not everybody feels the same amount of upset at similar events. Important factors are genetic predisposition; state of health prior to the upsetting events; social factors surrounding the event, such as social support; individual perception of the event; and physiological reaction to the event. This human complex makes the task of researchers immensely difficult, as does the retrospective nature of inquiry, for those who have had a heart attack are more likely to remember past life events than those who have remained healthy.

Life Events and Depression

Immediate stress from events like birth, illness, overwork, and loss may precipitate acute depression, while stagnation and boredom may lead to chronic depression. The birth of a baby can cause depression in both mother and father. In the mother it may be related to emotional stress or to hormonal changes. In the father it may be due to many different and unexpected emotional reactions to the child, to the change in family lifestyle, or to the increased financial burden. Acute depressive reaction following the death of a loved one is almost universal. However, repression of grief may also lead to long-lasting depression. Grieving openly is not encouraged in Western society, and failure to grieve can lead to prolonged numbness and depression.

Depression may follow marriage, divorce, separation, children's leaving or starting school, a family quarrel, or the illness of a close family member. It is not unusual to have mixed feelings about these events. Difficulty in expressing those feelings can lead to depression. Worries about work and money matters are often not expressed openly, and repressed feelings not only drain us of energy but also lead to depression. Failure to face up to difficult changes in life, like menopause or retirement, can lead to depression.

Brown and Harris (15) from New Bedford College in London have carried out a lot of work on the relation between life events and depression, and they feel that to quantify stress by just adding up the score of life events is too simplistic. It is not a particular life event per se but its meaning to the person concerned that is important. For example, a woman who really wants the baby is much less likely to be stressed by a pregnancy than the woman whose pregnancy is unplanned.

Below is a list of events which commonly occur in life. In the right-hand column there are stress points. Higher points mean the likelihood that higher stress is created by that event. Write down the stress points in the left-hand column if the event has occurred in your life in the last twelve months.

EXERCISE: HOLMES AND RAHE SCHEDULE OF RECENT LIFE EVENTS

Event	Stress points
Death of spouse	100
Divorce	73
Marital separation	65
Jail term	63
Death of a close family member	63
Personal injury or illness	53

Marriage	50
Fired at work	47
Marital reconciliation	45
Retirement	45
Change in family member's health	44
Pregnancy	39
Sex difficulties	39
Addition to family	39
Business readjustment	39
Change in financial state	38
Death of a close friend	37
Change to different line of work	36
Change in number of arguments with spouse	35
Taking out a large mortgage or loan	31
Foreclosure on mortgage or loan	30
Change in work responsibilities	29
Son or daughter leaving home	29
Trouble with in-laws	28
Outstanding personal achievement	28
Spouse begins or stops work	26
Starting or finishing school	26
Change in living conditions	25
Revision of personal habits	24
Trouble with boss	23
Change in work hours or conditions	20
Change in residence	20
Change in school	20
Change in recreational habits	19
Change in church activities	19
Change in social activities	18
Taking out a small mortgage or loan	17
Change in sleeping habits	16
Change in number of family gatherings	15
Change in eating habits	15
Holiday	13
Christmas season	12
Minor violation of the law	11

Total score   ____

What does the score mean?

Less than 150	30 percent probability of developing an illness, i.e. no more than average risk.
Between 150 and 299	50 percent probability of developing an illness.
Over 300	80 percent probability of developing an illness.

One of the problems of such predictive measures is the possibility of their becoming self-fulfilling prophecies. The purpose behind them, however, is not to notify us of the probability of becoming ill but to encourage us to take preventive measures.

3

Personality Factors or Behavior Patterns

In medicine it is often disputed whether the personality or behavior pattern of an individual has anything to do with the causation of organic disease. The reason is partly that the possible contributing behavior is much further in the past than the usual risk factors and therefore the connection is difficult to make, and partly that the physiological mechanisms linking the two are often obscure or must be observed for many years. Nevertheless, many believe that personality or behavior traits are critical in the chain of events which leads from excessive stress to the development of specific stress-related disorders. When life events cluster and the level-of-stress score is high, these personality or lifelong behavior patterns are important determinants of how that stress is likely to manifest itself.

Nowhere has the stress-prone personality been studied in greater depth than in association with coronary heart attacks. Many astute physicians and psychologists of the past have observed relevant and often profound details about the personality characteristics of individuals who are prone to coronary heart disease (142). In 1768, William Haberden added to his vivid description of angina pectoris: "The disease is created by the disturbance of the mind" (142). John Hunter, a nine-teenth-century English surgeon from St. George's Hospital in London, is reported to have said, "My life is at the mercy of any rascal who shall put me in passion." He proved his point by suddenly dying during a heated discussion at a boardroom meeting (142).

An American physician, William Osler, was asked in 1910 to deliver a series of lectures based on his extensive experience with angina and heart attack patients, about fifty in all. (Compared with 160,000 deaths per year due to heart disease in England and Wales alone in recent years. Coronary heart disease was rare then.) Osler had studied his patients carefully, and he described the coronary-prone person as one "who is keen and ambitious, the indicator of whose engines is set full speed ahead" (97). K. A. and W. C. Menninger (89) described such people as frequently exhibiting an aggressive personality. H. F. Dunbar (28) sized them up as hard-driving and having goal-directed behavior. C. Kemple (65) described the coronary-prone person as an aggressive, ambitious individual with an intense emotional drive, unable to delegate authority or respon-sibility with ease, having no hobbies, and concentrating all his thoughts and energy in the narrow groove of his career. S. G. Wolf (143) described him as one who not only meets challenges by putting out extra effort but also takes little satisfaction in his accomplishments. Dr. Henry Russek and colleague (116, 117) remarked on the striking degree of self-control, the dig-nified reserve, and the complacent exterior.

TYPE A BEHAVIOR PATTERN AND HEART DISEASE

Two cardiologists from San Francisco, Meyer Friedman and Ray Rosenman (36) have done extensive work in this area. They described an overt behavior pattern and called it "Type A behavior." The individual with this behavior pattern is portrayed as intensely ambitious, hard-driving, competitive, having a sustained drive for achievement, impatient, having a keen sense of time urgency, constantly preoccupied with occupational deadlines, involved in a chronic struggle to achieve as many things as possible in the shortest possible time, and, if anybody or anything gets in his way, likely to become aggressive and hostile. This hostility is often very well rationalized. Those who show these characteristics are designated Type A, those who do not show these characteristics are designated Type B, and those who do not strictly belong to either category are often classified as belonging to Type X. A further differentiation is often made between those who are ordinary and those who are extremes of Type A and B as A1 and A2 or B1 and B2. Although the reference is often made to Type A's being a personality, it is not strictly a personality type, which is much more a part of our intrinsic nature and not modifiable. Rather, Type A is a constellation of behaviors manifested under stressful circumstances by susceptible individuals.

There is an interesting story behind how Friedman and Rosenman began to conceive their ideas about the Type A behavior pattern's being linked to heart disease. Soon after they started their joint practice in San Francisco, they had to get an upholsterer to repair their waiting-room chairs and sofas. The upholsterer asked the receptionist, "What kind of patients do these doctors treat?" When the receptionist inquired, "Why?" the upholsterer remarked that only the edges of the chairs had been worn out; the patients seemed to have been sitting on the edge of their seats as if unable to relax. At first, the cardiologists didn't take much notice. In 1956, however, when studying the dietary habits of a group of upper-middle-class women and their husbands as part of their research into heart disease, the president of the women's organization commented, "If you want to know what is going to give our husbands heart attacks [heart attacks occur more frequently in men], I will tell you. It's the stress they have to face in their business, day in, day out. Why, when my husband comes home at night, it takes at least one martini just to unclench his jaws!" (See Friedman and Ulmer, 38). Friedman and Rosenman took these observations seriously and have since carried out a number of studies to show that the Type A person is indeed more liable to get heart attacks than the Type B person.

Type A can be measured by using an interview technique developed by Rosenman in which an interviewer who is more challenging than sympathetic is used. Sometimes the interviewer asks questions in a slow, deliberate manner to see if the respondent jumps in to finish off a sentence because of his impatience. The technique has recently been developed into a videotaped interview. During the scoring of the interview, the individual's speech style and mannerisms are also studied. Explosiveness of voice, restless mannerisms, and taut facial gestures, for example, are given high scores.

At first, Friedman and Rosenman and their colleagues showed that Type A individuals have raised cholesterol and triglyceride levels—the types of fats which are implicated in the development of atherosclerosis, or the hardening of the arteries. They also showed that blood from Type A individuals clotted much more quickly and that there was a greater release of stress hormones in response to challenge. The best known research is the Western Collaborative Group Study, in which the investigators classified 3,154 men aged 39 to 59, mainly white-collar upper- and middle-class executives working in the San Francisco Bay Area, by using the interview technique, and followed them up for eight and a half years. The death rate from coronaries was twice as high in the Type A group as in the Type B group (114).

It is often thought that Type A behavior is a coronary risk factor only for middle-class, white American men. However, in a second large study carried out in the town of Framingham, Massachusetts, Haynes and Feinleib, using a self-administered questionnaire, classified both men and women in white-collar and blue-collar jobs as well as housewives and followed them up for over ten years (50, 51). Again, Type A people were found to suffer an excessive number of heart attacks during the years of follow-up.

The Type A behavior pattern has been shown to be associated with excessive heart disease in Wales, in Japanese men living in Hawaii (20), in Belgium (67), and in Israel (86). In one British survey known as the British Regional Heart Study (63), Type A was associated with increased prevalence of heart disease, but it did not predict the development of an excessive incidence of new heart disease during the years of follow-up. In an American survey known as the MRFIT study (93), again the Type A behavior pattern did not predict excessive future risk of heart disease, but some critics feel that this might have been the case because the people chosen for the research were already at high risk because of high blood pressure, high levels of blood cholesterol, and cigarette smoking and because extensive attempts were made to modify their lifestyle and reduce the risk by means of drugs and diets. With individuals already known to be at risk it would be morally difficult not to try to change their behavior, and therefore it is unrealistic to expect their behavior scoring to predict future disease.

Despite some positive associations, it is difficult to accept that merely being ambitious and hardworking is harmful. In order to be more specific, Karen Matthews and her colleagues (82) reexamined the interview tapes of those who had suffered heart attacks in the Western Collaborative Group Study, comparing them with the interviews of those who had not suffered heart attacks, and found that the characteristics which differentiated men who had had heart attacks from those who had not were all related to anger and hostility, while rapid movement, hard driving, and being involved in one's job were not.

More recently, Friedman and his colleagues recruited over one thousand heart attack victims and randomized them to a treatment group, which was offered cardiac counseling and modification of Type A behavior, and to a control group, which was offered cardiac counseling only. During four and a half years of follow-up, only 12.9 percent of the treatment group, compared with 21.2 percent of the control group, had a recurrence of heart attack—a significant decrease (37a).

Main Characteristics of Type A Behavior

There are two main characteristics of the Type A person: a sense of time urgency and hostility. These are based on the original hypothesis of Friedman and Rosenman. Recent observations have indicated some uncertainty about these characteristics, and some think that either hostility alone (4, 26) or with competitiveness is the damaging ingredient (83, 84), but we have to bear in mind that only the original hypothesis has been tested in long-term studies, and therefore what is described here is Friedman and Rosenman's original viewpoint.

1. *Time urgency.* This is the feeling that there is not enough time to do all the things that we believe should be done or that we wish to do. It leads to the following symptoms:

- Rapid movements: The afflicted person usually walks, talks or eats fast. There is a dislike of dawdling at the table after eating.
- Impatience: There is a feeling that the rate at which most events take place is too slow. Frequently there is an attempt to hurry the speech of others by saying very quickly over and over again, "Uh huh, uh huh," or "Yes, yes, yes," or interrupting before people finish their sentences. There is anguish at waiting in line or waiting to be seated in a restaurant. When necessary but repetitive tasks have to be performed, like making out bank deposit slips, writing checks, and washing and cleaning dishes, the Type A person will try to avoid them.
- Indulgence in polyphasic thought or performance, that is, thinking or doing two or more things simultaneously, such as thinking about other matters when conversing

on the phone and not giving the other person undivided attention. Similarly, using an electric razor when eating breakfast and dictating a letter when driving a car both stem from that sense of time urgency.

- Tension: The Type A person finds it difficult to sit and do nothing. He feels quite guilty when relaxing. He often has a characteristic facial tautness expressing tension and anxiety.
- Restlessness: The restless body and mind are reflected in mannerisms like knee jiggling, rapid tapping of the fingers, head nodding, rapid eyebrow lifting while speaking, sucking in air while speaking, expiratory sighing, tongue-to-front-teeth clicking during conversation, or tuneless humming.
- Preoccupation: The Type A person is inattentive to others. He is unable to detect mental and physical fatigue while engaged in a task. He fails to observe the more important, interesting, or lovely objects encountered in the social milieu, so he does not enjoy life. Because of preoccupation with things worth having, there is not enough time to become something worth being.

2. *Hostility.* As used in this context, *hostility* is defined as a durable predisposition to evaluate people or events negatively, often in a suspicious, distrustful, cynical, and paranoid fashion, while anger is an emotional complex incorporating feelings ranging from minor annoyance to rage and fury. There is a generalized aggression or excessive competitive drive. These are reflected in the following symptoms:

- A habit of explosively accentuating various key words in talking, even when there is no real need for such emphasis. Speaking in an explosive, staccato, frequently unpleasant-sounding voice.
- Playing any type of game (even with children) to win.
- Clenching the fists, pounding the table, or forceful use of the hands and fingers.

- Challenging another Type A person, rather than feeling compassion for his affliction.
- Preoccupation and irritation with the trivial errors of others, including irritation with the drivers of cars in front who are running at a pace considered too slow or with other behavior of drivers.
- Being excessively critical of oneself and others.
- Characteristic facial expression of aggression, hostility, and struggle, as well as ticlike drawing back of the corners of the lips, almost exposing the teeth and habitual clenching of the jaw or grinding of the teeth.
- Irritation or rage when asked about past events which previously caused anger, as there is a tendency to relive the past.
- Tendency to swear or use obscene language.

Causes of Type A Behavior

Friedman and his colleagues believe that Type A individuals have certain tendencies which make them behave in certain ways. These tendencies are as follows:

- *Insecurity.* Excessive self-protectiveness even at a cost to other members of the team. Avoiding taking action rather than making a mistake, especially if being evaluated. Unable to delegate for fear of losing control.
- *Reactive modus operandi.* Crisis mode of operation. Believes he works better under pressure. Chronically underestimates time required for a task.
- *Touchiness.* Overly sensitive to and defensive about criticism.
- *Egocentricism.* Dominates conversations. Is interested in self only (narcissistic). Has difficulty in refraining from bringing conversation round to self-interest.
- *Suspiciousness.* Distrusts others' motives.

- *Competitiveness.* Belittles achievements of others in efforts to feel superior. Perceives other group members as adversaries.
- *Resentment.* Harbors feelings of ill will toward others.
- *Prejudice.* Has stereotyped generalizations about groups.
- *Deterministic worldview.* Believes self to be a pawn of the environment, rather than active determiner of fate.
- *Short-term perspective.* Deals with problems from the view of immediate consequences.
- *Belief in inherent injustice.* Acts like the policeman of the world.
- *Impatience.* Belief that success has been due to the ability to get things done faster than others, and fear of ceasing to do things faster and faster.
- *Perfectionism.* Believes, "I can do it best so I will do it." Unable to delegate authority.
- *Punctuality.* Has a fetish about being punctual.
- *Tendency to be critical.* Ruminates over a past mistake. Considers a "pat on the back" self-indulgent. Tends to look down on other people's inadequate performance.

The most comprehensive psychological explanation of why Type A people respond to perceived challenges or threats as they do has been provided by Dr. David Glass of New York University and his colleagues (41, 42). In his view, Type A behavior is a coping response used to counter the threat of actual or potential loss of control. Whenever signs of possible loss of control occur, as they frequently do in our changing environments, the initial Type A response is increased effort to regain control, involving greater mental and physical exertion, a stepped-up pace, and competitiveness. Thus the Type A person spends enormous energy in his constant pursuit of his achievements while maintaining control over his environment.

Even when control is not possible, the Type A person tends to deny this and continues to struggle harder and harder. He fails to recognize, emotionally or physically, that he is going full speed ahead and thus permits himself to keep working and struggling until he drops. When absence of control becomes obvious, the Type A person falls into a state of collapse. The reason is that he is not aware of fatigue or other signs of physiological and psychological stress when he is fighting to keep control. Since he is unaware of his tension, he does not take any steps to alleviate it until he has given up the fight in a state of helplessness. Thus the usual pattern of Type A coping style is one of aggressive hyperresponsiveness interspersed with depressive hyporesponsiveness (108).

A second hypothesis relating to the Type A behavior pattern, put forward by Larry Scherwitz and his colleagues is the excessive self-involvement of Type As compared with Type Bs (119). According to Virginia Price, there is a constant comparison between the self and the ideal self and further striving to reach the standards of that ideal self. When the goals of the ideal self become unattainable despite trying hard, the Type A person becomes depressed. Sooner or later he manages to drag himself out of that depression by becoming angry. Anger releases stress hormones like epinephrine and norepinephrine and helps to lift his depressed mood. Once out of depression and into the angry mode, the Type A person makes superhuman efforts to reach the goals of the ideal self until he is depressed again; the cycle continues until finally he is exhausted (108), which is usually when he suffers a heart attack. Karen Matthews and J. M. Siegel have also studied the Type A behavior pattern in children and suggest that the development of Type A behavior is encouraged by high standards of achievement subconsciously imposed by adults, particularly parents (84).

TYPE B BEHAVIOR PATTERN

Main Characteristics of Type B Behavior

- Absence of all habits and traits listed above that harass the severely afflicted Type A person.
- Absence of the sense of time urgency and its accompanying impatience. Does not make unrealistic commitments.
- Absence of free-floating hostility and lack of need to display or discuss achievements or accomplishments unless such exposure is demanded by the situation.
- Plays for fun and relaxation, not in order to display superiority at any cost.
- Able to relax without guilt, and to work without agitation.
- Cooperates with others. Gives the benefit of the doubt to others instead of imagining the worst.
- Flexible; can be either a leader or a follower depending on the situation.
- Generally respectful of others' integrity. Not afraid to admit mistakes. Gives others credit when due.
- Encourages trust and openness in team efforts.
- Delegates authority as much as possible.
- Takes a break when fatigued.
- Not devastated by criticism; "Tell me more" attitude.

Summary

- Research indicates that the Type A behavior pattern is associated with an increased propensity to get heart attacks.
- The Type A person is hard-driving, competitive, and impatient, with a tendency to become irritable and aggressive.

BEHAVIOR TEST

Circle the number which you feel closely represents your own behavior

Casual about appointments	1	2	3	4	5	6	7	8	9	10	11	Never late
Good listener	1	2	3	4	5	6	7	8	9	10	11	Anticipates other (nods, interrupts)
Never feels rushed	1	2	3	4	5	6	7	8	9	10	11	Always rushed
Can wait patiently	1	2	3	4	5	6	7	8	9	10	11	Impatient while waiting
Casual	1	2	3	4	5	6	7	8	9	10	11	Goes all out
Takes one thing at a time	1	2	3	4	5	6	7	8	9	10	11	Tries too many things at once, thinks what to do next
Slow deliberate talker	1	2	3	4	5	6	7	8	9	10	11	Emphatic in speech (may pound desk)
Cares about satisfying oneself,	1	2	3	4	5	6	7	8	9	10	11	Wants good job recognized

no matter what others think											
Slow in doing things	1	2	3	4	5	6	7	8	9	10	11	Fast (walking, eating, etc.)
Easy going	1	2	3	4	5	6	7	8	9	10	11	Hard driving
Expresses feelings	1	2	3	4	5	6	7	8	9	10	11	Hides feelings
Many outside interests	1	2	3	4	5	6	7	8	9	10	11	Few interests outside work

How to Score and What the Score Means

On each item you can score a minimum of 1 point and a maximum of 11 point. If you add up points on all the items you can score a minimum of 13 points and a maximum of 143 points. Most people fall somewhere in between.

104-143 = Extreme Type A
91-103 = Type A
65-90 = Type B
13-64 = Extreme Type B

Note. Adapted from Bortner, R. W. (1969). A short rating scale as a potential measure of pattern behavior. Journal of Chronic Diseases, 22: 87-91.

- In a population, those with existing heart disease are seven times more likely to be Type A than Type B.
- Type A individuals are more than twice as likely to get acute heart attacks as Type Bs over a period of follow-up.
- Type A personality increases the likelihood of a second heart attack.
- Research has shown that Type A behavior is modifiable.
- Modification of Type A behavior reduces the chance of further heart attacks by almost half

PERSONALITY PATTERNS AND CANCER

Is there a particular personality or emotion complex which predisposes people to getting cancer? It is doubtful if a clear-cut cancer personality exists. However, there is some evidence that cancer patients are likely to have suffered severe emotional disturbance in early childhood (anytime up to the age of 15). This may be due to the loss of the relationship with the parents, perhaps due to divorce, the death of either parent, chronic friction between the parents, or illness in one of them leading to prolonged separation from one or both parents. As a child he has usually suffered a great sense of loss, loneliness, anxiety, and rejection.

In order to overcome the feeling of failure to form warm and satisfying relationships in childhood, these people make special efforts to overcompensate by trying constantly to please others and win their affection. If they don't succeed, they feel further loneliness, anger, helplessness, and self-hatred, and eventually anxiety and depression become their constant companions. However, because of their extraordinary efforts to win affection in later life, their friends often describe them as most gentle, thoughtful, kind, and considerate. Despite this "good as gold" label, underneath many potential cancer patients feel worthless and hostile and dislike themselves, but most of these emotions are suppressed.

During adulthood, most cancer-prone people manage to gain a measure of success in love and healthy relationships through career, marriage, and/or parenthood. For the first time they feel genuinely happy and optimistic. As this happiness is dependent on external factors, some loss in life, such as the death of a spouse, the loss of a job, or children's leaving home to make their own nest, makes them feel desolated and they are once again drowned in their sorrow and depression. Sometimes within six months or a year of this loss of significant other person or thing in life, cancer appears. Their despair deepens when cancer is discovered, and they are back into the helpless-hopeless mode of living again.

The hypothesis that certain individuals may be psychologically predisposed to developing cancer is not, however, new. The ancient physician Galen observed in 537 B.C. that melancholy women were more likely to suffer from cancer than sanguine women. Eighteenth- and nineteenth-century physicians noted that a common thread running through all cancer victims was a reaction of despair and hopelessness following such diverse occurrences as the death of a friend or relative, separation, and economic, political, professional, or other frustrations. They lost all desire to live, and by virtue of this type of passivity, the stage was set for the development of malignancy.

Once established, emotional stress can stimulate the rate of malignant growth. A psychologist from New York, Lawrence Leshan, studied 250 cancer patients quite intensively through questionnaires and long personal interviews and concluded that four factors differentiated the cancer patients from a control group: (1) a lost relationship prior to the diagnosis of cancer; (2) an inability to express hostility in their own defense; (3) feelings of unworthiness and self-dislike; and (4) tension over their relationship with one or both parents. Some form of childhood traumatic experience was present in 62 percent of the cancer patients compared with 10 percent of the control group (69). Caroline Thomas and Karen Duszynski studied 1,337 medical students between 1948 and 1964 with extensive psychological testing and followed them up for a number of years in order to identify the personality patterns of those who are predisposed to suicide, mental illness, malignant tumors, hypertension, and coronary heart disease; they found that the group who developed malignant tumors had a distinctly distant relationship with their parents (137).

Harold Voth, a psychiatrist at the Menninger Foundation in Kansas, examined many patients and studied the medical records of numerous other cancer patients. He suggested that there is a strong relationship between the development of cancer and a melancholy, anxious disposition accompanied by continued low-key depression and a limited capacity to cope with life. He noted that most victims had suffered a "significant emotional loss" up to five years before the onset of the disease. A specific life event may not be as important as the person's reaction to that occurrence (106). Personality factors determine how an individual will react, and that reaction can be healthy or pathogenic. But although certain predispositions may be established, they are not thought to be irrevocable.

Dr. Carl Simonton, a cancer specialist in radiotherapy, and his psychologist wife, Stephanie Matthews-Simonton, along with James Creighton, have done the most innovative work in the psychological treatment of cancer patients. Drawing on their clinical experience, they described cancer patients as having (1) a great tendency to hold resentment and a marked inability to forgive; (2) a tendency toward self-pity; (3) poor ability to develop and maintain long-term relationships; and (4) a very poor self-image. They believe that psychological, emotional, and personal belief factors play a very important part in the onset and course of malignancy. They help their patients to alter the course of their disease through the development of positive psychological attitudes and through creative visualization. For example, a cancer patient is helped to develop a mental picture of cancerous material being destroyed by the body's immunological system, which is further boosted by deep relaxation and meditation (127).

PERSONALITY PATTERNS AND MIGRAINE

Migraine headache is a result of disturbance in the tone of blood vessels over the head. Patients who suffer from migraine tend to exhibit many of the characteristics of the Type A behavior pattern described earlier. They feel the same sense of unworthiness that haunts Type A individuals, and they also try to accept a greater burden of work than they can effectively cope with. Their exaggerated need for love and admiration and the approval of others stems from their own feeling of inadequacy. However, the futility of this approach leads to frustration, anger, poor judgment, and, at times, sudden bursts of hostility.

Migraine patients can be rigid, somewhat self-righteous, and at times fanatical. They try too hard at everything they do and discriminate poorly between tasks which are of major importance and those which are less important, which either can be delegated to others or do not require such major expenditures of energy. Paradoxically, migraine attacks occur during periods of leisure time, as if the victim has bottled up all the emotions and frustration of work, to be afflicted when finally it is time to relax and unwind. One obvious difference between migraine sufferers and Type A individuals is their self-sacrificing nature. In order to win approval, migraine sufferers willingly take on more than they can deliver. Coronary-prone Type A individuals, on the other hand, are more aggressive in their achievement and performance and tend to be ruthless in their effort to master the environment and control the course of events. Kenneth Pelletier (106) suggests that patients who suffer from migraine have the initial psychological response of drawing back from emotional involvement. They literally cease to let their emotional expression flow out toward other people, and they begin to contain their anger and resentment. One of the effects of this habitual response, he suggests, is the typical cold extremities that migraine patients have at the start of an attack. If the emotional withdrawal continues sleep-onset insomnia may follow. This fits well at this stage, the author says, since the last place where migraine sufferers are likely to feel expansive is while sleeping in the same bed or room as the person they resent. Of course the insomnia could also be interpreted as a normal stress reaction initiated to maintain vigilance in a situation which is perceived to be threatening. After a period of disrupted sleep pattern, the classical migraine symptoms of nausea, sensitivity to light, and visual aberrations begin to appear.

PERSONALITY PATTERNS, RHEUMATOID ARTHRITIS, AND ULCERATIVE COLITIS

These conditions are known as autoimmune diseases in which the body "turns on itself." Researchers have wondered if a particular form of self-destructive personality translates into a self-destructive autoimmune disease. Drs. Moos and Solomon studied the histories of 5,000 patients with rheumatoid arthritis. The characteristics which differentiated rheumatoid arthritis patients from a control group were a tendency to be "self-sacrificing, masochistic, confirming, self-conscious, shy, inhibited, perfectionistic and interested in sport." Female patients with rheumatoid arthritis were nervous, tense, worried, moody, and depressed, and typically had mothers who rejected them and fathers who were unduly strict. They had difficulty in expressing anger and scored higher in the measures of inhibition of anger, anxiety, depression, compliance-subservience, conservatism, security-seeking, shyness, and introversion (91).

A classic study of ulcerative colitis patients by George Engel identified personality characteristics strikingly similar to those of patients with rheumatoid arthritis, involving an obsessive-compulsive behavior pattern, excessive neatness, indecision, conformity, overintellectualism, rigid morality, and anxiety. Like the sufferers from rheumatoid arthritis, they could not express hostility or anger directly and seemed immature and dependent. They generally had mothers who were controlling (32).

Given the similarities in personality factors and behavior patterns of patients who suffer from migraine or heart disease and those who suffer from rheumatoid arthritis or ulcerative colitis, it is clear that multiple factors, including genetic susceptibility, are involved in the determination of which specific disorder will develop. It is also important to remember that the findings are only suggestive. Moreover, the purpose of exploring these characteristics is not to alarm people who may exhibit some of the characteristics but to make them aware of their vulnerable mode of behavior and under what conditions it is likely to manifest itself. Only awareness can encourage us to examine our attitudes and psychological orientation and to take positive preventive steps by doing something about them.

HARDY PERSONALITY

Just as there are people who are excessively prone to stress, there are people who are extremely resilient. Scientists have been interested in studying the characteristics of these people too. A psychologist from New York, Suzanne Kobasa, and her colleagues studied different groups of people and described a behavior pattern which they called the "hardy personality." This is found in people who are likely to be resistant to stress because they have a disposition composed of the 3

"Cs": commitment, control, and challenge (66). They are committed to what they do. They find a sense of purpose and meaningfulness in their work, family, and social institutions. They know their values and priorities, which give them a sense of perspective and an ability to make accurate judgments and to resolve problems. They know they can depend on others and that others are counting on them. Aaron Antonovsky, and his colleagues, other prominent researchers in this area, also considered this sense of community and accountability to others the most fundamental interpersonal resource for coping with stress (1a).

These people have a tendency to believe that they can control or influence the course of events. They take responsibility for what they do and for what happens in their lives. They are able to incorporate unexpected events into an ongoing life plan and are generally flexible enough to be able to deal with whatever comes along. An alienated person, on the other hand, feels his life is being controlled by others. He lives by rigid rules, and if things don't go exactly as he expects, he gets anxious and stressed. The Type A person also believes in control but his view of control is quite different. He actually fears loss of control and therefore strives hard to keep control, while the hardy person is more confident and less anxious.

Resilient individuals view challenges as normal and as an opportunity for personal growth, rather than as a threat to security. They view challenges with a sense of adventure and are willing to explore new situations. They are resourceful people and know where to go for help. They have an open mind and are flexible enough to tolerate ambiguity.

4

Occupational Stressors

Most people spend the major part of their waking life at work. More often than not we are identified by the work we do: he is an architect, she is a professor of anthropology, he is an electrician. No wonder that we introduce ourselves by stating what we do for a living: work is a most valuable source of satisfaction, as well as of stress. What happens to us at work is important to our health and well-being. When we lose a job, it means far more than just losing a source of income. We lose essential contact with other people; there may be increased fatalism, low self-image, and a feeling of helplessness. Hans Selye suggested that work is a biological necessity (122). Another study found that job satisfaction was the most important determinant of recovery from a heart attack (147).

Job stress can undermine our sense of personal worth and dignity. Different administrative styles can stir up different kinds of unconscious conflicts within each member of a group. Different jobs are carried out by different types of workers—engineer, secretary, executive, or printer—yet everyone expects to get satisfaction from the particular job he performs. Nowadays workers are demanding an increasing degree of fulfillment as human beings. Work also provides the best refuge from a major loss or from problems which might otherwise be difficult to overcome. For a person in this situation, loss of his job would be equivalent to depriving him of the only possible means of coping with stress outside of work.

It is also becoming increasingly common for people to experience changes in their work pattern, either because of promotion or as a result of technological advances. It is learning to adapt to these changes that is likely to be most stressful, especially when changes occur too frequently or are perceived as a threat to a worker's comfort, freedom or satisfaction. If promotion is thrust upon a reluctant worker his morale will suffer, and if his new job demands skills for which he has no training, there will be strain. If, on the other hand, he has been striving for that promotion his motivation and creative drive to succeed will enable him to overcome many difficulties, and he will work harder and grow more mature. Sometimes resistance to change occurs because of lack of communication, which leads to uncertainty, confusion, or ambiguity about what the job entails. Sometimes people are expected to play conflicting roles.

The terms *work overload*, *time pressure*, *conflicting demands*, *uncertainty*, *underutilization of skills*, and *work monotony* are embedded in our culture. However, they do not invariably produce stress. On the other hand we may feel stressed although none of the above factors is operating. As stated earlier, stress is determined by external forces as well as by the internal state of the individual and his ability to cope with the specific demand. Moral support from a colleague can increase our internal resistance. Some organizations structure work patterns that allow flexibility and greater control over the environment and more opportunity to be creative. Thus the individual, his groups, the organization in which he works, and the environment in which the organization functions can all interact and contribute to his resilience or susceptibility. Breakdown occurs only when stressors exceed the capacity of the individual or the organization to adapt. If the individual's ability to cope has already been stretched by the existing stress a new stress may well tip the balance.

MANAGEMENT STRESS

The acceptable standard of management performance is continually rising, so the manager who barely keeps up with last year's standard and fails to learn new things will certainly be under stress (64). Most managers find that there is more demand on their time and resources than they are able to meet. Resolving new problems and questions, the daily work leaves them no time to plan and innovate or learn new things until everyone has gone home, when they can sit down and work uninterrupted. This work period is often extended into family life; catching up on reading literature or preparing reports can occupy evenings or weekends. Fast-moving, high-pressured business often means crossing time zones on long-distance flights, sleeping on hotel beds, drinking excessively and eating rich food, as well as separation from family, and all these strains can add up. Ever-increasing restrictions on financial resources add to the total burden of stress for managers who are trying to keep their heads above water to produce results under time pressure against all odds.

Competing for promotion may mean that managers have to play office politics in order to be noticed by their bosses. Some become rude and aggressive. A new position or a new job, particularly in a new company, exposes them to a high level of tension as there are no established routines and relationships to support and protect. If the boss has an abrasive communication style they may turn objective and possibly justifiable comment into a personal criticism. Personality conflicts with colleagues can lead to exchanges of words which are felt as damaging to their dignity, the most painful words they are expected to absorb. Fear of being fired, a feeling of falling behind in performance, the possibility of being made a scapegoat during crises, and the fear of exposing inadequacy may lead them to drink excessively rather than to seek expert help. When one feels trapped in a job; when the opportunity for alternative work is limited; when one is so dependent on the income that leaving the job, even temporarily, is out of question, then the job becomes an inescapable, soul-destroying burden.

Today the merger and amalgamation of companies is becoming more frequent. When one company is taken over by another, there may be a crisis of loyalties and identities, particularly when international and transcultural cooperation is required. When individuals who are hopelessly and permanently incompatible are required to work together, so many personal resources are wasted that potential creative abilities are hampered, and if no escape is found, health will suffer. More hidden than interpersonal conflicts are the internal conflicts which arise when people are required to do something against their better judgment or their conscience. Inevitably, some managers will suffer burnout.

WORKING-CLASS OR BLUE-COLLAR STRESS

Arthur Shostak, the author of *Blue-Collar Stress* (125), suggested four basic concerns of workers: pay, safety at work, the quality of the work setting, and the stability of the job. His interviews with workers suggest that despite higher absolute levels of pay, fringe benefits, and ownership of a greater number of consumer goods, they feel under greater stress. With regard to pay or rewards, workers are concerned with the struggle not to lose ground to inflation's erosion of purchasing power. Despite overtime and the contribution made by a greater number of working wives and older children, economic unease continues to grow. When inflation and taxation are taken into account most workers fall into the bottom half of the wage-earners' pile. In most countries that practice market economy inequality in pay between those on the lowest rung of the ladder and those on the highest has been widening in recent years.

Unfortunately, the steps necessary to keep up with inflation, such as increasing pay demands, not only are likely to increase inflation further but the lower-grade workers can only fare worse compared with their higher-grade counterparts in management. In addition, they feel uncomfortable for being blamed for the wage-price spiral and for losing competitiveness in the international market. There are no golden handshakes or hellos for these people and no private pension scheme, private health insurance, company cars, expense accounts, business lunches, or spouses accompanying them on business trips. Things are made worse by intergroup rivalries, "no strike" deals by other unions, and fights to maintain pay differentials between skilled manual workers on one side and semiskilled or unskilled workers on the other. Collective bargaining means that unions negotiate on behalf of all workers or the employer grants increases to all with no regard whatsoever for individuals' needs or merits. If a person makes nothing for himself, by his personal efforts, his personal significance, his incentive to better himself and his self-esteem are reduced.

As far as health and safety at work are concerned, accidents at work, in the United Kingdom, cost 23 million working days a year, while various forms of mental stress and illnesses cost a further 37 million working days. In the United States, over 14,000 workers die annually and over 100,000 workers are permanently disabled through industrial accidents. In addition media news about workers being exposed to hazardous chemicals and toxic fumes* increased workers' tension and anxiety, which also rob them of health and well-being.

---

*As many as 14 million workers are exposed to toxic materials, and perhaps 600,000 workers are already endangered from postexposure to cancer-causing materials.

Work settings and working conditions are important stressors. Physical discomforts like noise, odors, poor lighting, and poor ventilation are common. Working outdoors in extremes of weather or working indoors without proper ventilation increases the risk of illness. What upsets workers most, however, is the loss of dignity and pride resulting from management's indifference to workers' comfort and satisfaction. When there are obvious double standards of care for white-collar workers and shop-floor workers, jealousy is likely to ensue. Another irritation for blue-collar workers is rules and regulations which make them feel like robots. Regulations about where to park their cars, when to start work, when to stop work, when to eat, where to eat, what to eat, where to smoke, when to smoke, when to go to toilet, when to wash up, when to take holidays, how to work, with whom to work, and whether or not to stroll or stretch can cause aggravation and tempt workers to retaliation and sabotage, which only make the relationship with management harder and the rules stricter.

Psychological satisfaction from work is important to workers' sense of well-being but is often completely ignored. To quote the chairman of the 101st annual Trade Union Congress on why industrial unrest and strikes occur:

> Where work gives little satisfaction to the worker, where there is no freedom to exercise talent or skill, where men and women do not determine how they do their work, where they have become merely components in the production system, they have, during their working lives, lost their identity as individuals. . . . Nobody who has not experienced the effects of years of confinement within the walls of mass production, without apparent means of escape, can understand the debilitating effects on the mind, the vocabulary, on the spiritual capacity of human endurance. Nobody, without this experience, can really understand why men down tools, when on the surface there seems to be only a pretext, to escape momentarily from the monotony of an unnatural existence (64).

In a society where prestige hinges on degrees and qualifications, on giving orders rather than taking them, on clean self-paced brainwork rather than machine-paced manual work, blue-collar workers' social status is likely to be low. Pride in what we do or in ourselves is the most important antidote against stress, but among lower-grade workers only a tiny minority seem to have this pride. Unfortunately, technological advances which mean machines can perform tasks better than people undermine what little pride some craftspeople have left. This leads to antipathy toward their work and a preoccupation with material gain, which is totally inadequate to compensate for low status.

In most industrialized countries the average number of days lost through illness or accidents among unskilled manual workers is three to five times greater than among professional workers. The reason is not just that these jobs are boring and unpleasant or the workers are less responsible about their jobs; this circumstance also reflects a true difference in mortality between the rich and the poor—a gap which, contrary to expectation, has been gradually widening since the 1930s.

Fear of layoffs in the face of massive unemployment means continual suffering in silence. As the author of *Work Stress*, Alan McLean (77) puts it:

> Unemployment and the threat of job loss are exquisitely threatening to many; seriously disrupting to others. Job insecurity leads to suspicion of the management and sometimes counterproductive attitudes and behavior; sometimes fantasies of leaving the present job for a better and more interesting job which doesn't exist. Past experience of unemployment leaves workers looking over their shoulders, if it's going to be their turn next to receive redundancy notice.

Technological advances displace many semiskilled and unskilled manual workers from their jobs every day. This stressor takes a major toll on workers' equanimity. Alternative jobs may require further training or extreme interunion cooperation, as transferring to a different job protected by another union is not easy. As automation spreads, repeated firings are not uncommon. Frequent "failures" leave people feeling negative about looking for another job or using their initiative.

SHIFT WORKERS' STRESS

Productivity targets which necessitate the use of expensive machinery twenty-four hours a day to be economical inevitably involve shift work of varying cycles. Frequently changing shifts are stressful biologically as well as socially and emotionally. Biologically, it has been shown that normally there is a decrease in the excretion of hormones like epinephrine and cortisol, a fall in body temperature, a decline in performance, an increase in fatigue, and secretion of restorative hormones in the night, and a reversal of all these patterns in the early hours of the morning and during the vigil of the daytime. This circadian rhythm or biological clock cannot be changed instantly, although the body does respond slowly to environmental demands. A one-week cycle of shift work is not sufficient for complete adaptation to take place. Swedish researchers have shown that even three weeks of a cycle are not sufficient to cause a complete inversion of the circadian rhythm in most subjects. They studied several hundred shift workers by means of questionnaires and found higher frequency of sleep, mood, digestive, and social disturbances among shift workers than among day workers, the complaints reaching their peak during night shifts (71). Other researchers have found that the blood cholesterol and blood pressure levels of shift workers are also high.

Shift work is also stressful socially and emotionally. An Australian worker summed up his feelings as follows:

As a shift worker my world is an endless round of changing shifts in which personal and family life suffers most. The confusion of weekly changing shifts [and] sleeping and eating habits is further heightened by the often unfilled demands of a growing family. I have largely had to forgo the companionship of my sons while they were young, so that they now look outside the home for many of the things that I would like to give them. My wife, who has had to work during most of our married life, has also missed many of the social contacts which are necessary for a happy life. Unfortunately, the result has been that our family life has degenerated into an unreal existence of club life for my wife and myself and a street corner existence for my sons. The hopeless part of it all is that I have no particular skill and have to work shifts to maintain my present earning. . . . Another thing that bothers me is the thought that most of my fellow workers and myself are just "getting by" although we are living in a boom economy. If this is prosperity I wonder what would happen if the economy should level off or decline? (64)

UNEMPLOYMENT AND STRESS

Between 1945 and 1960 there was full employment in most parts of the United Kingdom. It was assumed that most people would have jobs for the rest of their lives. Today more and more jobs are disappearing as a result of technological advances, automation is rendering many unskilled jobs obsolete. It is a common human need to feel that what we do is useful to at least somebody. When one is unemployed it is difficult not to feel useless. If the period of unemployment drags on, life without a goal or function feels like life without a soul. It can create anger and bitterness, but this soon gives way to helplessness, hopelessness, and even severe depression. Unfortunately this feeling of depression can trigger a vicious circle because a depressed person does not feel energetic enough to seek work. Even if he manages to get an interview, his low mood will prevent him from giving a sparkling performance, and no employer wants to engage a person who is less than enthusiastic. Being rejected intensifies the feeling of hopelessness and uselessness, which can be compounded when individuals are surrounded by unemployed families, as can happen in some areas in these days of high unemployment.

In short, unemployment can be a living hell. Sociologist E. E. Le Masters (68) explains why:

- The men resent the fact that it was not of their own choosing and thus point to the lack of control over their own fate.
- They can get bored to the very edge of sanity.
- They tend to drink more when they are not working. Le Masters says, "Many of these men have what might be called 'a drinking problem' which they control, at least in part, by not drinking on the job eight hours a day, five days a week. Unemployment upsets the delicate balance of their working program partly because they spend more time at the tavern when they are not working."
- Their marriage may become unstable as their wives are not used to having their husbands under their feet all day. "The husband, being upset by his inability to work, is not, of course, at his best in his marital role during this period."

The financial squeeze can be excruciating. Unemployment benefits help but the gap between unemployment compensation and active earning is hard to accept—particularly when the person is not to be blamed. Le Masters concludes that "one of the best indicators of the importance of the job to these men is their discomfort when they can't work."

STRESS AND THE WORKING WOMAN

In 1906 the tsar of Russia received a petition from some peasant women complaining about the fate of women. The author of "Women's Improved Role" cites (146):

> For generations the women of the peasant class have lived without having any rights whatever . . . we are not even considered human beings, but simply beasts of burden. We demand to be taught to read and write, we demand that our daughters be given the same facilities for learning as our sons.

Today a majority of doctors and teachers in Russia are women. Women account for three-quarters of cultural workers and two-thirds of all economists in the country. Of those working in science, 40 percent are women. A similar trend can be seen in other countries. In 1960, 35 percent of American women worked. By 1980 this percentage had increased to 51. New Zealand was the first country to give women the right to vote in 1893. Between 1917 and 1920 women in Russia, Great Britain, the United States, and Canada earned the right to vote. They had to wait longer in other countries.

Two world wars have contributed greatly to women's emancipation. Today we see women in senior posts, as eminent scholars, and as capable politicians. The number of women working outside the home has more than doubled in the last twenty-five years. In 1970 women held 27 percent of office jobs. In 1984, 65 percent of office jobs were held by women (146). Many women work because of economic necessity; some work out of choice.

Despite these breathtaking achievements there are still some amazing inequalities. Legally speaking, a woman has the right to earn the wage as a man doing the same job, but in practice there are many exceptions. Although there are more women voters than men voters, only three of the fifty state governors are women, and only thirty women have a seat in Congress. Despite legislation for equality of opportunity, very few top administrators are women. Unescorted women are not allowed in certain men's clubs and in restaurants where single men can enter with pride. Facilities like credit cards, mortgages, rentals, or bank borrowing are particularly difficult for women who are single, widowed, or divorced. In religion, women are not allowed to hold high positions such as bishoprics or archdeaconships. And there has been a price to pay for what women have achieved.

For example, there is the familiar conflict between pursuing a career and rearing a family. One newspaper report stated that women executives in the United States are far less likely to give their home life a high priority than their male peers and are twice as likely to be single or divorced. Men look at their home environment as a support system while women see it more as a burden. When a man comes home he sits in his armchair and relaxes; that's what he has been working for. For the woman, however, the second workload starts as soon as she comes home. One study reported that a woman with preschool children who has a forty-hour-a-week job outside the home works an average of seventy-seven hours a week. Those extra thirty-seven hours are spent doing household chores: cleaning, cooking, shopping, laundry, ironing, caring for the children, and other tasks. While women have expanded their responsibilities, they have not been given extra help in their traditional roles. The same study reported that the amount of time husbands spend doing housework has increased by less than thirty minutes a week in the last ten years (113). Some studies have shown that men are helping more than that; however, male attitudes and behavior have largely remained unchanged.

Many women cope with their tension and overwork by excessive eating, smoking, drinking, and medication, all of which damage their health further and drain them of vitality. Dr. Holly Atkinson, the author of *Women and Fatigue* (2), suggests that not only is the nurturing role burdensome in itself, but the conflict between playing the traditional role and developing an independent career outside the home is even more exhausting. Women are constantly at odds with themselves, trying to perform both the roles. Even though women's aspirations, hopes, expectations, and ideals have changed and their education and abilities in all fields have put them on a par with men in many, their unconscious minds have not kept up. Traditional images of what women should be and how they should behave have been imprinted in their minds since childhood, and these clash with their newer images of free, emancipated, fulfilled women. This hidden conflict leaves them utterly drained and exhausted. A woman's traditional voice shouts "guilty" when she leaves her baby with a babysitter each morning, sends her son to a boarding school, or admits her senile mother to a nursing home. It cries "fraud" in the face of success, demands a higher standard of housework, and labels her "selfish" when she takes time off for herself. Such constant pulling and pushing makes endless demands on her emotions and time.

In addition to carrying the dual load, women also have to put up with physiological disadvantages. Many women suffer from premenstrual tension, when the body and mind show signs of stress. They are more jittery, accident-prone, and likely to make rash decisions, and the quality of their work may suffer. Yet how often do their employers or family make allowances for their physiological state?

Similarly, no allowances are made for women who suffer menopausal symptoms. Through their sexuality and power to reproduce, women have been made the executors of the greatest miracle of this world: the creation of new life and the sustenance of the human species. In some countries this special role has been recognized to some extent and women continue to receive pay during the last weeks of pregnancy and a few months after the delivery, but this provision is not universal. Even in the most affluent country in the world, the

United States, I was saddened to see a physician wife having to return to work six weeks after her baby was born. These six weeks' leave were not maternity leave. She had worked throughout her pregnancy and saved her four weeks of annual leave; two weeks were added as sick leave. To top it all, she still had to make up the nights and weekends on call she had missed when she returned to work.

Women are further tormented when they have to divide their loyalties between work and the welfare of their children, especially when the children are sick. At all times they need to be fed, washed, clothed, taken to school, and given a chance to get ahead in the world. Some fathers share these chores, but they remain primarily the mother's responsibility. Similarly, caring for aged or disabled parents or relatives is a woman's responsibility, for which she is never adequately rewarded.

No wonder women feel tired. A sustained majority of women managers complain of tiredness as their main symptom of ill health. When I was a general practitioner, the most common complaint I heard from women was "Doctor, I feel tired all the time." On the surface it may seem ironic that the more labor-saving machines women have, like washing machines, dishwashers, microwaves, and vacuum cleaners, the more tired they seem to get. The reason is that women have taken on a new burden of working outside the home without relinquishing the old responsibilities in the home. As a result they are simply overworked and underappreciated, while conflict between the new demands and the traditional role is psychologically draining. In the face of such problems, it is no wonder that some women lose their femininity or sensitivity.

One of the most successful women on Wall Street stated, "Work to me is recreation. I like what I do and I make very few concessions," and this includes her family. Her two children are looked after by her businessman husband. Her associates described her consuming interest as "clearly not good for family relationships." This state of affairs is not applicable just to executive women. Women who are clerks in stores also find that working outside the home as well as caring for the family is a burden. The general expectations of our society are that women are the heart of the family and must be warmer to create the atmosphere of warmth and love. Thus society expects women to carry a double load, while many husbands fail to share in the domestic chores. Many wives outstrip their husbands in earning capacity and professional status and many husbands find this difficult to accept and adapt to. This creates emotional distance between the couple, often creating a crisis in the marriage and even divorce.

If crime is the result of social unrest and injustice, women certainly seem to be sharing a large part of it. Between 1974 and 1979, the number of women arrested for fraud in the United States rose by 50 percent compared with 13 percent among men. Embezzlement by women increased 50 percent while for men the increase was only 1.5 percent. Forgery and counterfeiting arrests among women rose by 27.7 percent compared with 10 percent for men. Smoking has been declining in men but continues to rise in women. If deaths from lung cancer in women continue to rise at the present rate, it may replace breast cancer as the number one cancer among women. Alcoholism in women is also not infrequent.

The fact that a career or job does not give all the satisfaction a woman wants is revealed by Megan Marshall in her book *The Cost of Loving* (80). She says that, "the facade of professional competence only thinly concealed the private wounds: disappointed loves, compulsive promiscuity, lesbian experimentation, abortions, divorce and just plain loneliness."

More women than men complain of psychosomatic symptoms and symptoms of mental illnesses like anxiety state and depression, but they still live longer. Why? It could be that they release their tension by these means, and that by getting earlier medical attention they manage to prevent serious illness. Social science research has also shown that women have more positive and trusting attitudes and they smile 50 percent more than men. In addition, having to play so many roles in life—wife, mother, cook, cleaner, home economist, family nurse, and chauffeur, as well as wage earner—makes women more resilient than men in general. Thus, despite inequalities and social injustice, women will generally survive stress better than men.

WHO SUFFERS?

It is often believed that the higher a person's position at work and the greater the responsibility he has, the more likely he is to be stressed. Medical evidence suggests the contrary. A study of London civil servants (78) showed that mortality from heart attacks among lower-grade employees, like messengers or clerical assistants, was three and a half times greater than among top-grade administrators. Studies from American insurance companies confirm this observation, showing that the death rate in company presidents is only 58 percent of the country's average of all men of the same age. It may be that the challenging tasks they carry out have positive rather than negative effects and that they derive a greater degree of satisfaction from their job. When jobs are boring, repetitive, or monotonous, they provide insufficient mental stimulus and stifle creative energy. Lack of control over the work environment is another source of work stress.

EXAMPLES OF OCCUPATIONAL STRESSORS

- Change in work practice requiring new skills
- Numerous deadlines
- Lack of feedback from the top about job performance

- Responsibility without adequate authority
- Unclear goals
- Boss with abrasive communication style
- Lack of communication about serious problems in the company
- Lack of leadership in times of crisis
- Poor design of work process
- Inadequate rewards—low salary, poor prospects
- Threat of being fired
- Lack of clarity about the scope and responsibilities of the job
- Hostile customers
- Trapped in an unsatisfying job
- Lack of control over the work environment
- Incompetent co-workers
- Transfer involving geographic relocation
- New management style
- Technological change
- Too many meetings
- Divided loyalties
- Lack of stimulation at work
- Boredom and monotony
- Job without meaning
- Too much work and too little time
- Insufficient time to do job properly
- Equipment breakdowns
- Lack of privacy
- Insubordinate juniors
- Little opportunity for learning new things
- Frequent night shifts
- Conflicting demands
- Unclear line of authority
- Mistrust of those in power
- Changes from above imposed without consultation

EXAMPLES OF PHYSICAL AND PSYCHOLOGICAL ENVIRONMENTAL STRESSORS

Physical

- Unsuitable chairs
- Desk too high or too low
- Noisy surroundings
- Poor lighting
- Poor ventilation
- Uncomfortable uniforms
- Unbearably hot or cold atmosphere
- Unhygienic conditions
- Toxic fumes
- Odors
- Precision work causing eye strain
- Handling dangerous material
- Standing, walking, or bending all day
- Lack of regard for safety regulations

Psychological

- Office politics
- Sarcastic remarks
- Hostile atmosphere
- Isolated environment
- Overcrowded environment
- Sexual harassment
- Pessimists
- Indecisive stallers
- Bullies
- Silent, unresponsive types
- Smokers
- Loudmouths
- Superagreeable types

- Gum chewers
- People who are rude
- Moaners and groaners
- Know-it-all experts

5

Domestic Stressors

MARRIAGE OR PARTNERSHIP

When two individuals, with different family backgrounds and established relationships, decide to live together for the rest of their lives, there are bound to be some changes. Marriage, to be successful, requires a series of adjustments by the partners, as well as the establishment of accord, intimacy, and commitment. Adaptation to any change invariably causes some stress. There is a constant process of adjustment, sometimes by one partner, sometimes by the other, as understanding deepens about each other's ambitions as well as intellectual and emotional needs and drives. However, there are bound to be times when there will be some differences. For the most part these differences are ignored. When other pressures appear, however, suppression of these differences, whether conscious or unconscious, cannot be maintained. Such irritations are not infrequent but more often than not they are recognized as mere irritations and accepted by the parties concerned. New and unfamiliar circumstances increase uncertainty and anxiety. A strong, supportive relationship between partners and their families can make uncertainties tolerable and can make successful adaptation easier. On the other hand, critical events may hopelessly break an unstable marriage.

In the past, when marriages were difficult to dissolve, the legal and domestic framework supported the partners while they made their adjustments. Gradual changes in the traditional roles of men and women have exerted a different kind of stress. Many women go out to work before and after having children. This wage-earning capacity makes them financially independent while eroding the traditional role of the man as "breadwinner." Some men feel stressed by this. Some housewives feel trapped by their biological role of bearing and bringing up children and unhappy about the fact that their potential in the workplace is not being fulfilled. On the other hand, they feel guilty if they decide not to have children in order to further their career. On the whole marriage protects men but does not offer any special benefit to women. In one study in California by Lisa Berkman and Leonard Syme (10) it was found that unmarried men were three times more likely to die early than married men, while for women, being married or single did not make any difference. Further research carried out in Framingham, Massachusetts (29, 51), has shown that a wife's educational background and the type of work she does also have a bearing on the husband's health. It was shown that men married to women with a college education (a total of thirteen years or more of education) were 2.6 times more likely to develop coronary heart disease than men married to women with only a secondary-school education (a total of eight years or less). Men married to women in higher jobs were three times more likely to develop heart disease than men married to clerical workers or blue-collar workers or to housewives.

On the whole, men tended to marry women with similar educational, family, and social backgrounds. Although a less frequent occurrence, men with secondary-school education who married women with higher education were 4.4 times more likely to develop coronary heart disease. Most of these women in higher jobs were, however, teachers, nurses, or librarians rather than executives, professionals, or managers. Further exploration of the husbands who developed coronary heart disease revealed that their highly educated wives were significantly more likely to have a nonsupportive boss than those highly educated women whose husbands did not develop coronary heart disease over the thirteen years of observation. Thus it would seem that the frustration of a poor work environment is transmitted to the home situation and to other members of the family, just as stress resulting from disappointments in domestic life affects the quality of work and accentuates work stress (3).

Men who developed coronary heart disease in the above study had wives who were significantly less ambitious and more likely to report anger symptoms. This lack of ambition among wives was most significant for blue-collar men who developed disease. On the surface this seems odd and appears inconsistent with the previous finding that men married to highly educated women were more likely to develop coronary heart disease, as we would expect higher status women to be more likely to be ambitious. Contrary to expectations, blue-collar working women were more likely to be ambitious than either white-collar or clerical women. Women with some college training were the least likely to be ambitious, a finding suggesting that ambitions were already fulfilled among women who had achieved higher education.

Marriage does not, however, protect women as it does men. In fact, it may surprise you to know that the highest rates of distress are found in married women. Married women who do not work outside the home have the worst mental health. Studies have shown that, in general, employment has a positive effect on the mental health of women by improving economic status, increasing self-esteem and social contacts and alleviating boredom. Historically speaking, men have held power and authority and women have been rewarded for such psychological traits as submissiveness, compliance, helplessness, and passivity, which accommodate and please men. Modern women are struggling to break away from this traditional role and its injustices and to find new roles of independence and personal growth that raise self-esteem. Such struggles consume energy and leave them feeling drained.

The Subpanel on the Mental Health of Women of the President's Commission on Mental Health documented (18) the ways in which women's inequality creates dilemmas and conflicts for women in the contexts of marriage, family relationships, reproduction, child rearing, divorce, aging, education, and work. These same conditions of subordination also set the stage for extraordinary events that may heighten women's vulnerability to mental illness. The frequency with which incest, rape, and marital violence occur suggest that such events may well be considered normative developmental crises for women.

Many women feel out of control because they are constantly attending to the needs of others—spouse, children, aged parents, and so on. While she is busy nurturing others, caring for them and pleasing them, a woman rarely gets nurtured herself. While men consider themselves special human beings, confronting the world as a place to be mastered, conquered, and controlled, women lose their identity to the needs of others and eventually end up overworked, unfulfilled, and emotionally drained. Even if a woman is not physically overworked, boredom, low self-esteem, and inner turmoil frustrate her and rob her of all creative energy.

So what is the answer? Do women have to choose between family or career? The life consisting of all family and no work or no family and all work, or for that matter the life of conflict between the two, is an unbalanced life. We need both love and work in a harmonious proportion that boosts our energy and happiness and makes us healthy and productive. Even when both partners have independent and fulfilling careers, work interests may still clash. Who should subordinate whose career prospects when a job transfer or new prospects demand relocation? Many other conflict situations can occur. In a partnership, as in any other close relationship, emotions are intense and inevitably lead to frustration, dissatisfaction, and resentment. Such frustrations and anger require expression. All too often this expression takes the form of arguments and quarrels, which may clear the air but at a price. When feelings are repressed they lead to chronic and festering resentments. Long-hidden conflicts underlie many psychosomatic illnesses.

Conflicts may be about roles. For example, the wife may feel that she would like her husband to share in the domestic chores. The husband's macho image may be hurt by this expectation. There may be conflicts over spending and savings, who uses the family car, who decides which TV program to watch, where to go for holidays, who is right and who is wrong. Some people are so strongly opinionated that they are reluctant to put their opinions to the test. Standing up for our rights may be useful when dealing with injustice at work but being overassertive in a partnership or marriage can cause unnecessary conflict. We may win an argument but the end result may be the alienation of the whole family. We need to learn the art of constructive communication and dignified compromise. Harboring chronic resentments or grudges only leads to further stress.

Sexual difficulties may be another source of conflict. One partner's needs and tastes may be quite different from those of the other. Lack of communication about such matters may cause further dissatisfaction and nagging stress. If stress leads to premature ejaculation or impotence in the man and frigidity or loss of libido in the woman, relationships are further strained and tension increases. Unfaithfulness of one partner is a well-known cause of marital discord, often leading to divorce or permanent separation. Marriage counselors and sex therapists frequently remark on the incredible lack of communication between couples. Even those who have been married for years find it difficult to discuss certain things. Some subjects are still considered taboo, and frank discussion about them causes embarrassment. Even among the sexually emancipated, discussing such a subject is not always easy sailing.

Children can be a source of conflict as well as joy. Effective contraception gives women a choice of having or not having children. Such freedom in itself imposes responsibility and stress and can arouse conflict between partners. The prospect of having a baby may cause different reactions in the couple; one may be delighted while the other may become anxious. Whether or not there is a conflict, one thing is certain: there will be a loss of freedom with the arrival of a new baby. When the infant is sick there are not only further anxieties about its welfare but also the stress of lost sleep, having to stay home to look after it, and the possible loss of income which comes on top of an already increased financial responsibility. The husband may behave oddly because of the diversion of his wife's affection to the baby. Further worries may arise if the child misbehaves or does not do well in schoolwork.

Stress, whether it arises in or out of marriage, makes people behave in strange ways. Irritability or hostility may take the form of physical violence. Wife battering and baby battering are forms of assault resulting from aggressive impulses. Then there are changes in parental roles when children start school, leave school, take up jobs, and move out of the nest. As the menopause approaches, a woman's change of mood or behavior may give her spouse another problem to cope with. Individuals vary considerably but a quarter of women may need to make profound psychological and physiological adjustments, and these can affect the entire family. The male climacteric is less well defined but nevertheless exists. Further adaptation comes after retirement from work, or as the result of old age, disability, or the death of a partner. The death of a spouse is generally accepted to be the most stressful event that we can experience. It makes extraordinary demands on our ability to adjust to a new life, and many die of a broken heart.

Marriage or partnership is never plain sailing but for some it may unfortunately be very stormy. Some eventually have to face divorce or separation.

DIVORCE OR SEPARATION

The ease with which a divorce can be obtained and the growing feeling that a marriage is not necessarily for keeps can lead to the destabilization of a marriage and the dissolution of a partnership under stress. However, the process of divorce can be very prolonged and the path strewn with difficulties, not only legal and material but also emotional. It is unlikely that a divorce can be free of tension, conflicts, apprehension, sadness, regrets, or pain. Before accepting that the marriage is over, there is a phase of disbelief that this could happen. Partners are likely to alternate between hope and despair. The partner who feels rejected and unloved and who is agreeing reluctantly to separation is likely to feel anger as well as sadness, more intensely than the one who is the prime mover. However, things are never simple and the rejector is likely to feel on many occasions that he or she is being rejected or to have doubts about whether he or she should have tried harder, while the "innocent" partner may become ridden with guilt. The feeling of being the condemned and aggrieved party is likely to apply to both the partners at some stage or other.

Apart from sadness, the lives of both will be dramatically disrupted. Relationships with friends and family have to be renegotiated on the basis of a new social identity; financial apportionment has to be made; and most painful of all are the implications for the children of a marriage. In terms of stress score, divorce ranks second only to bereavement according to the Holmes and Rahe Life Events Scale. However, some of those who have experienced both feel that divorce can be more desolating than widowhood, which can at least be accepted as God's will. Bereavement also invites more sympathy and more support from others, while a divorce carries with it a sense of failure, guilt, recrimination, rejection, shame, humiliation, and responsibility.

In addition to loss of the partner, sexual intimacy, and companionship, a divorce can also involve the loss of day-to-day contact with the children, perhaps the loss of a house and a particular lifestyle, and most of all, the loss of hopes and aspirations. A lot of adjustment is needed before the feeling of loss and emptiness can give way to a new meaning in life. It has been suggested that after bereavement such an adjustment takes two years while after a divorce it takes five. The reason for such a long-drawn-out period of adjustment is the continuing attachment to and sense of connectedness with the former partner which prevents the establishment of a new life and equilibrium.

The legal process of divorce can be emotionally draining. Sometimes one partner uses a lawyer merely to force the other partner to discuss the issues. If the lawyer is perceptive, he will refer the couple to a counseling agency; otherwise, the matter will regrettably go too far and the couple will reluctantly reach the point of no return. Such a misfiring inevitably leads to anger, which can be displaced onto other problems, like the apportionment of money or property, and there may be prolonged disputes over the custody of children or access to them.

Being preoccupied by their own hurt ego and insecurity, parents may forget that continued conflict can seriously affect their children and behave like children themselves. Sometimes couples deliberately prolong disputes in order to avoid facing grief and emptiness or communicating the news to the children. However, children are extremely perceptive and leaving them out of the dispute when they already sense their world falling apart can be very stressful to them. Some adjust to the fact of separation or divorce relatively easily while others show severe behavioral disturbance. Their school performance may deteriorate and they may get into trouble with the police. Some children will try very hard to get their parents to stay together. The children's suffering is likely to further increase the stress of the couple. Divorce or separation of parents is undoubtedly a traumatic event for children and they will need reassurance and unqualified love from both parents. They are likely to cope better if the subsequent relationship between the ex-partners remains reasonably amicable and if they are not required to take the side of one or the other parent engaged in acrimonious conflict.

It is usually only with professional help, strong support from friends and relatives, and personal determination to overcome the pain and anger by expressing emotions and by making appropriate adjustments that the conflicts and problems associated with divorce or separation can be resolved.

EXAMPLES OF DOMESTIC STRESSORS

Marriage

- Lack of communication with spouse
- Difference in mutual interests
- Recurrent financial problems
- Sexual difficulties leading to frustration
- High unmet expectations
- Different values and priorities leading to conflict
- Different sleeping patterns through habit or nature of working life
- Spouse who snores
- Spouse who is overweight
- Irrational jealousy
- Unfaithfulness
- Deciding on leisuretime activities where interests conflict
- Sharing domestic chores

- Spouse's smoking and drinking habits of which the other disapproves
- Spouse's being away from home too much
- Lack of compliments
- Conflicting careers
- Illness of spouse
- Prolonged separation

Children

- Sleep disturbances due to crying infant
- Sick child who may be left with permanent impairment
- Disobedient children
- Jealous siblings
- Temper tantrums in shops or in front of friends
- Not having enough time with children
- Handicapped child
- Lack of respect for parents
- Having to love and look after stepchildren
- Food and clothing likes and dislikes
- Transporting children to schools and other places of activity
- Conflict between own and children's interests
- Child who plays truant
- Poor academic performance
- Lack of respect for teachers
- Bad behavior at school
- Children with untidy rooms
- Children playing loud music that drives parents mad
- Youngsters monopolizing the phone when parents are expecting an important call
- Late-night parties with ashtrays and broken glasses left for parents to pick up
- Children in trouble with police
- Children with drug problems

- Teenage daughter who gets pregnant
- Changing work ethics of the young
- Generation gap
- Incest

Other Domestic and Social Stressors

- Deciding to marry or not
- Single-parent family
- Divorce
- Aging parents
- Demanding in-laws
- Unplanned pregnancy
- Deciding to have or not to have children
- Relatives with unreasonable expectations
- Sharing gardening, house decorating and other chores
- Difficult neighbors
- Sharing house with relatives
- Alcoholism in the family
- Drug abuse in the family
- Domestic violence
- Serious illness in the family
- Aging
- Chronic illness
- Physical disability

6

Economic, Political, and Social Stressors

ECONOMIC AND POLITICAL CLIMATE

The climate created by national and international economic, political, and social changes may be harmful in itself. Even if these changes do not directly concern the individual, they can often sensitize him or make him more susceptible to other stressors. A recent example has shown us how the U.S. balance-of-payments deficit can drastically affect share markets around the world and the value of various currency exchange rates. Some may lose fortunes overnight in share dealings, and many others may be affected by interest rates or possible inflation or recession. Even those who do not feel directly threatened may be subtly affected by the change in value of their pension or insurance funds.

Contemporary economic and political problems affect the attitudes of workers, their confidence, and the quality of their performance. A change in public spending policy may lead to an increased burden in social cost as a result of unemployment. Greater affluence and a gradual rise in the general standard of living in the West have led to higher expectations and an insatiable consumer appetite. Massive imports of cheaper goods from developing countries may lead to further unemployment. Increased unemployment resulting from a variety of causes can herald racial tension and an increase in the crime rate. On the one hand, society and workplaces are changing fast; on the other hand, the bureaucratic machinery of government, industry, the police, education, and indeed the medical establishment remains resistant to change and insensitive to the needs of the people they served. Over a period of time minor problems and daily annoyances can add up and leave the individual in a very vulnerable state.

Productivity and efficiency are still the overriding values of our society today and hence health is implicitly defined as the capacity to help produce. This is why only lip service is paid to the importance of the health of the unemployed, aged, or disabled, who cannot sell their labor in the market. Many industries employ doctors, not usually for altruistic reasons but to keep the workers physically fit and to make it difficult for workers to "choose" to be ill—which is often their only defense against the stress and alienation of factory work.

SOCIAL AND ECOLOGICAL ENVIRONMENT

Only recently has awareness grown of the impact the social and ecological environment has on our mental, emotional, and physical well-being (27). It is beginning to be accepted that disease does not occur in isolation but is a manifestation of disharmony in our relationship to the universe. In folk medicine, religion, medicine, and morality are frequently intertwined, but today medical doctors consider themselves scientists who believe only in what is measurable and they focus on the basis of illness. It goes without saying that modern medicine has proved enormously successful in fighting organic diseases, particularly infections, and this success has helped to prolong our life expectancy although this extended life expectancy could not have been achieved without certain hygienic standards also becoming part of our everyday life. However, these achievements are used by most contemporary doctors to justify their refusal to alter the traditional view of illness.

Since the majority of illnesses that doctors have to face today have no detectable organic cause, we should at least be open to a revision of the traditional view of illness. That social and ecological factors contribute to health and disease is shown by the different distributions of various illnesses according to social class, religious or ethnic group, degree of industrialization, work situation, group affiliation, urban or rural living, the specific role played in the family, and socialization processes to which children are exposed. Besides, the expectations of contemporary patients are changing. Their complaints often include lack of an inner development, lack of creative energy, poverty of spirit, a feeling of meaninglessness, and a vague sense of uneasiness or malaise. These do not fit into our existing model of disease and we must therefore broaden our concept of health and illness to include psychological, sociological, economic, and political factors.

In a well-known study of 1,800 workers of the New York Telephone Company, it was found that 30 percent of the subjects suffered 70 percent of the illness. Those in the high-illness group were predominantly single women living at the parental home, who had to look after aged or ill parents and who experienced chronic dissatisfaction with their low-grade status in life (54). In a study, reported by Brown, of schizophrenic patients discharged from the hospital, it was found that a successful outcome, measured by remaining out of the hospital for at least twelve months, depended not on the severity of the symptoms but on the social environment to which the patients were discharged (14).

In a study of a large population by Thomas Holmes (55) in the city of Seattle it was found that for whites the occurrence of tuberculosis (TB) in both men and women was highest in the poorest and lowest in the wealthiest areas. However, for nonwhite populations the trend was reversed. The highest TB rates were among the people living in the richest area. These were professional or "successful" people of minority social groups who had been pioneers in moving into previously all-white areas. The investigators suggested that the restricted social interaction and the strains of living in uneasy social surroundings which resulted from differing values, upbringing, language, and skin color had a great deal to do with the higher incidence of TB.

The investigators also found that those developing TB were highly mobile people who had moved from place to place and job to job. They were more likely to be unmarried, divorced, or widowed, often living alone in furnished rooms. The author summed up their characteristics as follows: "They are strangers in the neighborhood in which they live. . . . They don't belong, they have few friends or neighbors with whom they interact, frequently, they have little family or kinship relationships and are generally restricted in social contacts."

Social Class and Health

Dr. George James (61) has reviewed the health crisis of the poor and cites one study in which it was found that the majority of men rejected by the U.S. armed forces for physical reasons were from poor environments. A real indicator of social injustice was the fact that 50 percent of the white rejectees were receiving care for their condition while only 16 percent of the blacks and 10 percent of the Puerto Ricans were receiving care. The fact of the matter is that a comparatively larger proportion of blacks and Puerto Ricans have a low income and inadequate education; and they are more likely to be unemployed and living in overcrowded housing.

The poor seem to suffer more from every physical and emotional disorder known to humans, including cardiovascular disorders, rheumatic fever, heart disease, diabetes, cancer, prematurity, infant mortality, schizophrenia, dental disorders, arthritis, rheumatism, visual impairments, and general mental disorders. The incidence of disease and death from all causes increases as family income decreases. Despite the increase in prosperity of the United States as a whole the gap between the health of the rich and of the poor is unfortunately widening. Dr. Roger Hurley (59) has reviewed several recent studies from the United States and shown that 50 percent of serious illnesses in the population are not treated. Most of these are in poor people.

Adjustment to Change

We are constantly making adjustments as part of our efforts to maintain equilibrium in the face of changing environments, but questions are beginning to be asked: Adjustment to what? To racism? To hijacking? To terrorism? To religious wars? To a violence-ridden society? To poverty? To polluted air? To radiation leaks? To Third World crisis? Brickman questions whether it is proper for a psychiatrist to use the label *affective disorder* to describe a violently angry man living in a black ghetto. What purpose does it serve to call a dissatisfied youth who turns to drugs an *inadequate personality*, when he never had a stable home (13)?

Pollution

Polluted water, mainly in the Third World, is responsible for about three-quarters of the world's illness. It kills 25,000 people every day of the year, every year, through water-borne diseases such as typhoid, dysentery, and cholera. Richer nations have other problems. Exhaust fumes from industrial plants, cars, and other transport and the domestic combustion of fossil fuels combine to change the actual composition of the earth's atmosphere. The gases released from burning fossil fuels and other pollutants are warming the earth through the greenhouse effect. Most scientists agree that by 2030 the climate will be warmer than ever before, with serious consequences as a result of a rising sea level and changing rain patterns.

Another hazard we are constantly exposed to is the ever-increasing quantity of chemicals in our environment, the toxicity of which is often unknown. Lamont Cole of Cornell University (21) stated that DDT was sprayed over the entire surface of the earth before we understood its noxious implications, and had it not turned out to be as harmless as it did life on earth could have come to an end. The U.S. Food and Drug Administration estimates that we are now exposed to well over half a million different chemicals in our environment, and the number is increasing by a thousand new chemicals every year. In the case of 80 percent of these chemicals we do not have sufficient information on their safety or toxicity.

Between 1 and 10 percent of all cancers are now regarded as being due to synthetic chemicals. This may be just the tip of the iceberg because it takes between twenty and forty years of exposure before the disease develops. Meanwhile more pesticides and other toxic chemicals are finding their way into our households and into our food and water. An unfortunate accident led to 3.5 million people in Britain drinking water with a higher level of aluminum (the metal connected with possible development of presenile dementia) than allowed by the European Economic Community; another 5 million drink water with an excessive level of nitrate, the compound some scientists think causes cancer. The thinning of the world's protective ozone layer by gases from aerosol cans, refrigerators, and hamburger cartons threatens to cause 40 million extra skin cancers and 12 million extra eye cancers over the next ninety years in the United States alone.

Women peace activists protesting outside the U.S. Air Force base at Greenham in England reported that some of their volunteers were having mysterious illnesses, including headaches, memory loss, nighttime hot flashes, menstrual irregularities, retinal bleeding, and miscarriage. They suggested that these symptoms indicated a health risk from exposure to non-ionizing electromagnetic radiation—the radio emissions and microwaves of long-distance communication systems and radar. Unlike the notorious dangers of the ionizing radiation of X rays and nuclear fallout, the health risks of microwaves, radiowaves, and extremely low-frequency (ELF) radiation have not been well established.

In the twentieth century petroleum replaced coal as the most important industrial fuel. The *Torrey Canyon*, a tanker carrying petroleum, was wrecked off the south coast of Britain in 1966, spilling a huge amount of oil. The Royal Navy and the Royal Air Force sprayed the areas with detergent. Later it was found that where petroleum, untouched by the detergent, had been washed up on the rocky shores, the marine snails went around cleaning up the shore. Apparently they could eat oil-contaminated vegetation without harmful effect, but where the detergent formed an emulsion with the oil the snails were killed and the mess was worse than if the detergent had not been used.

As stocks of fossil fuels run low we are turning to nuclear energy. Accidents like the one at Chernobyl remind us that radiation leaks are not just a frightening theoretical possibility but are actually happening. Overnight 50,000 people had to be evacuated, with very little hope of ever returning to their homes and roots. Such social disruption can have a devastating effect on generations to come in more than one way. Increased incidence of childhood leukemia in the neighboring population is already happening.

No illness has ever been eradicated just by treating the sick. Psychosomatic illness is no exception. Prevention, taking into account an ecological awareness of social and political structure, which helps the individual overcome his personal and interpersonal psychological and functional disorganization, must be given greater emphasis if we are to make a significant impact on stress-related disorders. Social institutions have to become more flexible and individuals need to be more resilient.

EXAMPLES OF ECONOMIC, POLITICAL AND SOCIAL STRESSORS

Economic

- Slow economic growth
- Recession
- Energy crisis
- Public expenditure cuts
- Reduction in productivity
- Balance-of-payment problems
- Reduced exports
- Increased imports
- Inflation
- Rising interest rates
- Consumer boom
- Devaluation of currency
- Rich-poor divide
- Unemployment
- Exorbitant house prices

Political

- Income tax
- Suspicions of those in government
- Stricter regulations
- Privatization
- Nuclear arms issues

- Education policy
- Bureaucracy
- Lack of leadership
- Dictatorship
- International tension
- Urban disintegration
- Corrupt government officials
- News media
- Strikes
- Hospital waiting lists
- Nuclear waste disposal
- Countryside preservation
- Wildlife preservation
- Pensions
- Welfare benefits
- Union power
- Immigration laws

Social

- Lack of morality
- Class discrimination
- Permissiveness
- Racial discrimination
- Overpopulation
- Human rights violations
- Social isolation
- Housing shortage
- Mismatch between numbers of eligible men and women
- Plight of the sick, old, and disabled
- Social outcasts
- Disharmony with neighbors
- Violence and hooliganism
- Domestic violence
- Drug abuse
- Drunken drivers

7

When Are Stressors Likely to Cause Stress?

Since most of us come across stressors every day, but only rarely get stress symptoms or illness, we must ask: When are stressors likely to be harmful? What makes people susceptible? In what contexts are symptoms most likely to appear? What seems to be important is the complex interaction between (1) types of stressors; (2) an individual's ever-changing susceptibility, and attitudes and beliefs; and (3) the social, political, economic, physical, and psychological environments in which stressors occur. If the social, psychological, and physical environments are optimum, and the person has a positive outlook, the person is likely to escape unscathed from the effects of demanding or challenging stressors. The robust individual may similarly remain intact despite demands and a pressured environment if his expectations are realistic.

Symptoms are likely to occur when all variables overlap or interact with each other. The factors are interrelated, each potentiating the others. Thus, too many stressors make the individual more vulnerable, and negative beliefs and attitudes or an uncongenial organizational climate may influence his ability to cope with everyday stressors.

WHAT MAKES US VULNERABLE

Our degree of vulnerability is constantly changing. Our constitution, family background, upbringing, education, previous experiences, present circumstances, mental attitude, ingrained beliefs, nutritional state, physical fitness, age, number of life events requiring adaptation, personality makeup, health habits, and biological factors all have a bearing on whether we will be successful in withstanding stressors or whether we succumb to them. We may not be able to change some of these factors but, if we can understand them, we can take better care to change those which are amenable to change and which are likely to tip the balance.

Ages and Stages of Life

Adolescence. Only those who are overly protected or very tough-minded sail through this stage without any stress. As the adolescent grows, matures, learns, and adapts to the special needs of this age, he or she has to cope with particular problems. There are physical changes of maturation to adapt to. There is a great deal of conflict between the need for emotional and intellectual freedom and the desire to remain a child and be protected. Sexual urges, tentative and unstable relationships with other adolescents, revolt against authority, or the sheer boredom of not having an independent role can cause considerable stress, which may be felt as minor anxiety or may show itself in the ugly forms of hooliganism, gang fights, pilfering, alcoholism, or drug dependence. Psychology and psychiatry texts devote a great deal of space to the problems and processes of the formative years and the maturation of personality structure in the teenage years and early twenties.

Early Adulthood. Personality development continues throughout life. Getting married, establishing a home, finding

a stable job, and raising children all take their toll in a multitude of stress symptoms and minor illnesses. Some of us are
lucky enough to have a fulfilling job, a stable marriage, and
domestic bliss, and youth still provides some resilience so most
young people are able to bounce back to health after minor
illnesses. Others are not so fortunate.

Midlife. Somewhere between the ages of 35 and 45 we
are suddenly faced with the reality that probably half our life
is over. Until now we were not too concerned about the future
as we were busy with our work and family commitments, and
old age seemed a long way away. Suddenly we realize that
time is not limitless and we can no longer afford to dream
about success. If we are going to succeed it is time for serious
action. Of course, if we have made our way in the world exactly as we wanted to or even better than we had expected,
this period in life, when we have the gift of greater maturity,
experience, and wisdom without significant loss of physical
strength, can be wonderful. But if we feel that we have failed
to fulfill our aspirations or an important part of our potential,
it can be very difficult to overcome the feeling that it is probably too late to start now and to hope to achieve our goal. A
feeling of lost opportunity and regrets at not having taken steps
earlier can be very depressing.

The period between ages 45 and 55 deserves special attention. The fear of aging, being over 40 and not knowing
where we are going in an organization, a change in the values
and the meaning of occupational and interpersonal relationships, and a change in our commitment to work, family, or
social institutions can be extraordinarily frightening. Midlife
crisis can affect anyone, irrespective of grade or rank, and
periods of depression are its most common symptom. The
person reaches a point where, perhaps after a struggle of "it's
now or never," his life is never the same again. Sometimes
people do rash things—divorce a spouse, change their job,

begin to drink or gamble heavily, or adopt a bizarre lifestyle. Men around middle age are particularly susceptible; some external or internal trigger can act as the "straw that breaks the camel's back." Coronary heart attack is one of the most common outcomes.

For women the menopause can bring more dramatic changes in life. The cessation of periods is sometimes accompanied by hot flashes, night sweating, vaginal dryness, and a number of vague symptoms like headaches, insomnia, digestive disturbances, breathlessness, weight gain, dizziness, and muscular aches and pains. The emotional changes can be very profound, and as many as one in five women feel moody, irritable, or depressed. Feelings about reduced femininity may affect a couple's sex life as well as create emotional distance between them.

Getting Old: 60 and Over. The time inevitably comes when we are reminded that we are getting old. Perhaps it starts when we need reading glasses, when we feel tired after shopping or physical work, when we feel a game of tennis is hard going, or when joints do not feel as supple as they used to be. The realization that life is moving on to its close may be very hard to accept, particularly the possibility of an illness or dependency and the certainty of death. As the body becomes stiffer and slower and arthritis sets in in many joints, the prospect of dependency becomes almost unbearable. Then there is the fear of losing friends, spouse, or close siblings; of becoming incontinent; of losing our memory; and of becoming a burden. Of course most people try to hide such fears, and such repression in itself can lead to depression.

Biological Factors

Biological factors which increase our risk of getting certain diseases are called *risk factors*. For example, high blood pressure, a high level of blood cholesterol (a type of fat), or dia-betes increases the risk of having a heart attack or a stroke. There is evidence that these are all in some way related to stress. Even if they are not caused by stress, they are certainly aggravated by it, and stress management programs can help to reduce their impact.

Although it may sound surprising, stress can actually in-crease the level of blood cholesterol independently of dietary factors. In a study carried out by Friedman and his colleagues (37) in the United States, a number of tax accountants had their blood cholesterol measured every two weeks. As the ac-countants got busier from January onward and as the April 15 tax deadline drew nearer, their cholesterol level started rising, reaching a peak just before the deadline. Once the deadline was met and work pressure began to lessen, the cholesterol level started to come down. Similar observations have been made by other investigators using different populations in pe-riods of stress.

In diabetes, the blood sugar level tends to be high. Efforts are made to control the level by diet or medication. Stress has frequently been shown to disturb this control despite continu-ation of the prescribed diet or medication. Many instances have been reported in which diabetes has been triggered, or first diagnosed, after a stressful situation like bereavement, an ac-cident, or a severe infection.

Unhealthy Lifestyles

Other factors which may reduce our resistance to illness are cigarette smoking, drinking too much alcohol, overeating or eating the wrong type of food, having a sedentary lifestyle, and being dependent on prescribed or nonprescribed drugs. The evidence is growing that smoking and alcohol, as well as other addictive drugs like marijuana, morphine, heroin, and cocaine, compromise our immune function and increase our susceptibility to serious illnesses, including cancer and possibly even AIDS. The immune system represents the body's defense mechanism, which fights invasion by foreign agents including bacteria, viruses, fungi, parasites, and even cancer cells. Once warned, the defense force marshals natural killer cells to seek out and destroy these foreign agents; the white blood cells send out tentacles that engulf and eat the invaders. B-cell and T-cell lymphocytes derived from the bone marrow and thymus gland, respectively (*B* and *T* stand for "bone marrow" and "thymus gland"), also play important roles. B-cells produce antibodies which combine with foreign agents to form antigen-antibody complexes which not only render foreign agents inactive but also trigger the complement reaction, which recruits at least nine serum proteins in the immunological battle. Complement enzymes burn through bacterial membranes, causing them to explode. Complement proteins also kill viruses. T-cells regulate and control antibodies.

Doctors have known for a long time that people who inject themselves with drugs like morphine are liable to get infections. Until recently it was thought that this infection was due to dirty needles, but recent evidence suggests an immunological factor which might be even more important. Morphine is known to depress immune function in mice and rabbits. Marijuana significantly lowers the amount of immunoglobulin G (IgG), which helps fight infections carried in the blood. Most of this knowledge comes from research on animals, and we have to treat the results with caution. Research evidence on humans is very scarce but it is accumulating.

You might remember a famous epidemic which occurred in Philadelphia affecting those who were attending a convention of the American Legion in 1976. There were 182 men who contracted deadly pneumonia, and 29 actually died. The cause turned out to be bacteria which were breeding in air conditioners. The name Legionnaire's disease was derived from the fact that the first known cases occurred in those Legion members attending the convention. Later it was reported that smokers had 3.5 times more risk of catching the disease than nonsmokers. A group of Australian researchers found that those who had stopped smoking for three months showed a rise in immunoglobulins and natural-killer-cell activity. It is known that alcoholics are more susceptible to tuberculosis, respiratory infections, and certain cancers. It has been reported that the majority of AIDS patients are drug users and it has been suggested that they get AIDS not so much through having sex with an infected person as from being already sick because they have a damaged immune system.

Unhealthy lifestyles and biological factors are interrelated. For example, overweight, consuming too much salt, excessive alcohol, excessive coffee, a sedentary lifestyle, lack of sleep, and stress contribute to the development of high blood pressure; cigarette smoking not only damages the lungs but also encourages atherosclerosis and, by making blood cells more sticky, also increases the risk of thrombosis. The usual Western diet contains more animal fat than is healthy for us. Such a diet tends to increase the blood level of cholesterol, which is implicated in heart attacks and strokes, which account for over half of all deaths in most Western countries. Individual factors which contribute to an unhealthy lifestyle are discussed in more detail in Part 2 of this book.

Attitudes and Beliefs

Not everyone responds to a potentially stressful situation in the same way. Some are able to take it in their stride, while others fly off the handle very quickly. The simple reason is that it is not the outside stressor alone that is important, but also how we interact with that stressor. We often have unrealistically high expectations. If we expect to win every contract, pass every examination, please every single person, or never make mistakes, we are demanding such perfect standards that we are bound to disappoint ourselves. Unresolved conflicts or unpleasant past memories, if allowed to run wild, will play havoc with the rhythm and equilibrium of our personal or work life.

Psychiatrists say that most fatigue stems from our mental and emotional attitudes. The emotions which drain us of energy are not the positive ones, like joy or contentment, but the negative ones, like resentment, the feeling of not being appreciated, and the feelings of futility, hurry, anxiety, worry, or frustration. These are the factors which exhaust many sedentary workers and make them susceptible to illness. We rarely get tired when we do things which are interesting and exciting for us. Even supposedly boring work, if we do it "as if" we actually enjoy it, may become enjoyable in reality and we can thus decrease our fatigue, tension, and worry. Thus our negative mental attitude is more likely to produce fatigue than physical exertion. Do you remember a day when everything went wrong and another day when everything fell into place and you really enjoyed the day? Which day was most fatiguing?

How are our beliefs and values formed? Who shapes our expectations and our attitudes? Most beliefs are formed in response to some need (75). For example, as children we need to be loved and approved by our parents. In order to feel safe and cared for we accept their beliefs about how to speak, how to behave with others, what is polite and what is rude, how to work, how to respond to pain or injury, what we can talk about and what is considered taboo, how and when to express sexuality, how to handle mistakes, what should be our goal in life, how self-reliant we should be, how much support to expect from our parents, relatives, or friends, and what our obligations are to family members and society in general. Such beliefs are promoted by the type of language our parents use, such as "Be considerate"; "Don't be rude"; "Always keep your dignity"; "Be generous"; "Education is very important"; "Don't let anyone push you around"; "If someone slaps you, slap back"; or "Always be kind to others irrespective of their kindness to you"; and so on.

As we grow up our beliefs are generated or modified by the need to win approval from our peers and the need to belong to a group. To ensure peer acceptance, we learn to live by the rules and beliefs of the peer group regarding how to handle aggression, how to behave toward the opposite sex, which political party is best, what we owe to society and the world at large, which type of health service is desirable, whether or not to fight for a cause, which cause is worth fighting for, and so on. If our friends oppose market economy, it will be difficult for us to support that system in the face of strong pressure to conform.

However, a number of studies have shown that values do change as circumstances and status change. For example, a prounion employee who fights for workers' rights may change his views, within months sometimes, once he is promoted to a management position and may even justify management beliefs and values. Again the need to belong and the need for safety create new patterns of belief so that we may fit in with the new group of which we are now a member.

A third major force in shaping our beliefs is our own emotional and physical well-being (76). The need to preserve our self-esteem, to protect ourselves from painful experience and loss, to enhance our pleasure, excitement, and the meaningfulness of our lives, and to feel physically safe are of paramount importance. Someone who is fighting an election for a high government office may ask his family for a self-sacrifice because he believes that once elected, he will be able to do a great deal for his community. It is completely irrelevant whether he really will be able to do much or even a little for the community. The reality does not matter as long as he believes that the position for which he is fighting is worthwhile, as well as bringing pleasure, excitement, and status. Our beliefs may stem from our need to maintain our self-esteem; if we get fired from our job we might say, "I was going to give up that boring, underpaid, soul-destroying job anyway."

If the family, culture, or society has inculcated the values that achievement is to be respected and lack of promotion is a sign of our own laziness, then it should not surprise us if we work incessantly to protect our self-esteem or feel dissatisfied if we do not achieve the standard we have set for ourselves. If, on the other hand, we, or our friends or parents, have repeatedly lost jobs despite hard work and honesty while the companies we worked for got bigger and more prosperous, it would be easy to become cynical and disenchanted with work ethics and to form the opinion that people are out there to exploit us or that hard work doesn't pay. In such a situation we would not feel guilty sending in a sick note for backache just to get away from the job for a few days.

If our life has been relatively easy and we have been surrounded by happy and jocular people, we are likely to develop a good sense of humor, but if on the other hand our life reads like a list of tragedies or we have been living with melancholy people it will be difficult to laugh and joke about ourselves. An unrewarding experience with a person of the opposite sex may make us believe that sexual relationships are more trouble than they are worth. If our parents or peers have criticized us every time we made a comment we are likely to become quiet and reserved and are likely to keep our mouth shut even though we are in a position to make a valuable contribution.

In summary, most beliefs and rules are formed in response to our needs and our past experience. We have learned them from our parents and peers and from our need to feel good about ourselves, our need to be loved and belong, and our need to feel safe. They have nothing to do with truth or reality, but the power of beliefs is such that we accept them as absolute truth or unbendable rules, not just for us but for the entire world. Such is the tyranny of "shoulds," write Matthew McKay and Patrick Fanning, the authors of *Self-Esteem* (76), that if we do not live up to our "shoulds" we consider ourselves bad and unworthy. That is why people torture themselves with guilt and self-blame, why they become paralyzed

when forced to choose between the "shoulds" they have in-
vented for themselves and their genuine desire.

The following list is of some of our "shoulds" and "musts,"
our unrealistic beliefs and our rigid attitudes:

- I should be in a higher position than I am.
- I should never quarrel with my spouse.
- I must never raise my voice to my children.
- I should be generous and unselfish.
- I should be a perfect lover, friend, parent, or student.
- I should be able to find a solution to every problem.
- I should have foreseen the problem.
- I must never be jealous.
- I should endure hardship with equanimity.
- I must not make mistakes.
- I will never be able to forgive myself if I fail.
- I should be completely self-reliant.
- I should not have relied on her to give me a lift.
- I must not indulge myself.
- I must take care of everyone who cares for me.

Obviously not all "shoulds" or "musts" apply to a single
person and not all values and beliefs are unhealthy. Of course
we must have values and priorities, provided that we don't
treat them as absolute truths. When we use words like *always*,
never, *ever*, *must*, *should*, *perfectly*, and *totally* we are applying such rigid rules that there is no room for a single mistake.
Striving for excellence is a worthy ambition, but not to be able
to tolerate an occasional mistake is setting ourselves a goal that
is impossible to attain. Realistic values lead to behavior which
results in a positive long-term outcome. "Shoulds" and "musts"
are unrealistic if followed blindly without any evaluation or self-
assessment. They require us to act on principle irrespective of
how much pain we may inflict on ourselves or others in the
process. Healthy values are flexible, modifiable according to
current needs, realistic, and life-enhancing rather than absolute,
global, unrealistic, and life-restricting.

We need to ask ourselves if our attitudes and values are really applicable to us. Our mother's belief that having a baby was God's will served her well in the absence of effective contraception, but to accept that ourselves without question may ruin our plans for a fulfilling career. Our father's belief in hard work may have been right for him but to follow that rule with our own angina may actually kill us. Not to express anger may have been appropriate in the gentle family we grew up in but it will take us nowhere in a cutthroat business world. Many of the values we grew up with may simply be out of date or not applicable to us in our present circumstances. Our old values should not become a consuming obsession.

Negative Self-Talk

Much of our stress is due to silent conversations we have with ourselves. Psychologists call this *self-talk*. We talk ourselves into the ground by programming ourselves negatively. Negative self-talk surfaces in our attitudes, beliefs, expectations, evaluations, interpretations, and predictions. When we blow things out of proportion by using words like *extremely*, *incredibly*, *always*, or *horribly*, we often come to believe in the things we repeat to ourselves. The tendency to put ourselves down is self-destructive. In fact, self-esteem and vulnerability are inversely related: when self-esteem is high, vulnerability is low, and vice versa.

Some people call this self-talk our *critical inner voice*. Everyone has this critical inner voice but people with low self-esteem have a particularly vicious one. It calls us names like *idiot*, *stupid*, *incompetent*, *lazy*, *failure*, or *screw-up* whenever we make the slightest mistake. It compares us with other people and their success or accomplishments and tells us that we will never get to that height of achievement because we are not capable. If we are less than perfect we are nothing. It exaggerates our weak points: "You are fat and ugly; how

can anyone ever like you?"; "You are so boring, you turn people off"; "You are so clumsy, you can never get anything right."
Such a sharp critic can be very damaging. We can get over
an illness or injury, we can even get over a great loss in life
in the course of time, but the critical inner voice is always
there, blaming us, judging us harshly, and hindering us in
everything we try to do. The nagging voice will somehow or
other manage to create doubt in our mind about our ability
to form a relationship or to do a good job or about the course
of action we have just decided to take. It makes us starkly
aware that we must be a real disappointment to our mother
because we chose to remain single or that our father must be
turning in his grave to see we have become a taxi driver instead of an engineer as he had hoped.

Why do we listen to this critical voice? The fact is that
it has become woven into the fabric of our thought. It has
become our second nature without our realizing it. We listen
to it because in some way it makes us feel safe and by raising
our defenses it prepares us for a possible defeat in the future.
If we have an adequate amount of self-esteem it will help us
confront challenges and solve problems instead of worrying
about them; we will make people respond to us positively
rather than blaming our luck; we will sort out interpersonal
problems as they happen instead of waiting for them to go
away or aggressively breaking up a relationship. If, on the other
hand, we happen to have low self-esteem, the critical inner
voice can make us safe in the face of challenges and interpersonal problems. It is better to accept defeat beforehand or to
blame others than to face the anxiety involved in confronting
things we are not sure about and to wait until the critical
voice tells us, "You blew it again. You just can't be trusted."
So if we say to ourselves, "I can never win" or "I always mess
things up," we will not be shocked if we do lose or things
turn out less than perfectly.

A temporary drop in anxiety or reduction in tension is so
relieving that such negative self-talk and behavior are further

reinforced. Unfortunately, negative self-talk really undermines our sense of self-worth. Another reason why the critical inner voice has such a strong hold on us is that there is still a part of us that is willing to believe that its approval, like that of our parents, is necessary for our survival. The critical inner voice is further reinforced when sometimes we do achieve things after it has driven us hard with vicious attacks on our competence and has whipped us like an old horse. Unfortunately such temporary gain is no match for the relentless stress it creates and the damage it does to our self-worth.

Chronic negative thinking is linked to poor health because our thoughts determine our behavior. Dr. Martin Seligman (120) and others have shown that animals faced with unavoidable electric shocks eventually give up trying to escape. Later, when they are put in a situation where they can easily escape by performing simple tasks, they do not even try because they have learned to become helpless. Many believe that in humans, too, a feeling of hopelessness leads to helpless behavior and even chronic depression. Seligman believes that even in the absence of a negative situation, mere negative thoughts generate helplessness. One failure in the past can lead to pessimism in those who are negatively predisposed. On the other hand, people who are optimistic and more positive may protect their bodies and minds from harm and may help themselves to live longer.

8

How to Recognize When You Are under Stress

EARLY WARNING SIGNALS

When the brain is exhausted it becomes difficult to concentrate and making a simple decision may seem like a big problem. If the feeling of tiredness is either neglected or suppressed by drinking alcohol or smoking cigarettes we may feel relieved but soon reach a point of diminishing returns. Thinking becomes muddled and if we continue to push ourselves we either become edgy and lose our temper or lose all perspective and feel completely hopeless. When feeling low, we may withdraw from social interaction. Sometimes people become moody and oversensitive to criticism.

Some people drink or smoke for enjoyment or to be sociable, but for others drinking or smoking is clearly a means of relieving anxieties or depression. A small amount of drink may help us to relax and reduce inhibition, and smoking a cigarette may lift the mood temporarily, but unfortunately both activities become habits and during stress we come to rely on them more and more. Consciously or subconsciously, cigarettes are lit and stubbed out in a chain and drink poured as if automatically, every time we feel under pressure or are irritable.

Eating patterns may change under stress. Some people go off their food while others turn to food for comfort. Losing or putting on weight can thus be a sign of long-term stress. Similarly, sleep patterns may change. Some are unable to sleep or have nightmares while others find that even a ten-hour sleep is not refreshing. Some clearly do not wish to wake up, while others cannot fall asleep because their minds are constantly riveted on the problem while their restless bodies toss and turn.

When angry, we are likely to rebel against rules and regulations and to become accident-prone. Chronic tension may result in all kinds of mannerisms like biting nails, pulling hair, and jiggling the knee. When the mouth is dry and the throat muscles tense, swallowing may become difficult and we may feel a sensation of choking. The muscles of the abdomen may be so tense that it feels as if the stomach is in a knot. Vomiting may be a sign that the person is unable to stomach something that is bothering his mind. Diffuse abdominal pain may be due to tension in the bowels, which may become constipated or loose. Similarly, the bladder may become irritable, the result being frequency of urination.

Our muscular system is held under finely tuned nervous control. During movements one group of muscles is taut while the opposing group is relaxed. Such intricate control allows manual dexterity and smooth execution of movements. During stress the fine nervous control is out of balance. Conflicting thoughts, so common during stress, are translated into alternative tension and relaxation, which lead to the characteristic shakiness of the hands and sometimes the whole body. Tremor of the vocal muscles shows in the characteristic trembling voice or stammering. Occasionally twitching may affect an isolated small muscle like the one at the corner of the mouth or eyelid.

Prolonged tension may drain the affected person of all energy. Mental tensions in a sedentary person may leave him physically exhausted. Of course people differ tremendously in their capacity, and hence the amount of work they can handle before feeling fatigued varies considerably, but it is important to recognize our own limit and to learn to take a break as soon as the limit has been reached in order to maintain vitality.

Lists of possible mental, emotional, physical, and behavioral signs of stress are given below. They are not specific, in the sense that sometimes they may occur for reasons other than stress. Some people are more likely to be aware of these symptoms than others. Therefore it is not necessarily the case that more symptoms mean greater stress. On the other hand, some people are so externally oriented that they are not in touch with their feelings. Such people deny having any symptoms but succumb to serious stress disorders like a heart attack. Only after suffering a crisis can they recall having been excessively tired before the event.

We respond to stress physically, mentally, and emotionally and in the way we behave. The physical signs are easy to understand when we understand the physiology of stress. Other signs are a little more difficult to recognize unless we are aware of them. Some of us respond predominantly through bodily symptoms, and others respond for the most part emotionally, but usually we show combinations of symptoms. It is important that we recognize the way we respond to stress. Unless and until we recognize our symptoms we will not be able to learn how to prevent or minimize them.

Examples of Mental Symptoms

- Inability to concentrate
- Difficulty in making simple decisions
- Loss of self-confidence
- Undue tiredness

- Memory lapses
- Difficulty in making rational judgments
- Undue feeling of being under time pressure
- Making rash decisions
- Muddled thinking
- Tendency to lose perspective

Examples of Emotional Symptoms

- Irritability or angry outbursts
- State of anxiety
- Irrational fear or panic attacks
- Feeling of hopelessness
- Feeling of hostility, resentment, or animosity
- Feeling of guilt
- Increased cynicism
- Undue aggression
- Feeling of depression
- Nightmares
- Feeling of insecurity
- Increased moodiness
- Crying or weeping
- Fear of criticism

Examples of Physical Symptoms

- Tense muscles (aching shoulders, backache, etc.)
- Erratic breathing
- Sweaty palms
- Cold fingers
- Dry mouth
- Dizzy spells
- Chest palpitations
- High-pitched voice
- Knot in the stomach

- Nausea
- Frequency of urination
- Diarrhea
- Stiff jaw
- Restlessness (e.g., pacing)
- Shaky hand

Examples of Behavioral Symptoms

- Increased smoking or alcohol drinking
- Increased or decreased eating
- Increased or decreased sleep
- Nail biting
- Hair pulling
- Social withdrawal
- Neglecting looks or hygiene
- Reckless driving
- Knee jiggling, finger tapping, grimacing, lip smacking, or other mannerisms
- Non-stop talking
- Obsessive-compulsive behaviors (checking locks, needless shopping or washing)
- Workaholism or absenteeism

Ask yourself what type of reactor you are. Are you mainly an emotional reactor or perhaps a physical reactor? Knowing the answer will help you to be aware.

STRESS AND ILLNESS

Persistent stress can lead to a variety of physical discomforts and serious diseases. Minor ailments like tension headache, migraine, backache, triggering of asthma, eczema, arthritis, palpitation, indigestion, diarrhea, constipation, and insomnia may not be life-threatening but can make us miserable and drain us of our resources. Major stress disorders like high blood pressure, heart disease, or cancer can indeed be life-threatening. Some of the common stress disorders and some steps which can be taken to relieve or prevent them are described below. Detailed accounts of how to reduce stress are given in Part 2 of this book. At this point, however, I wish to make it clear that there are also other causes of the disorders I have described below as stress disorders. To describe these other causes in detail is beyond the scope of this book. If you suffer from any of these ailments, you must see your doctor, who alone can tell you if there are other causes which must be treated by drugs or surgery. Stress increases our susceptibility to them and reducing stress can only be beneficial.

Tension Headaches

When muscles around the head remain tense for some time they may be felt as headache. An example of a situation requiring prolonged alertness or active use of muscles in this area is driving. Preparing for an important speech or having long arguments can lead to contraction of the muscles in the scalp, neck, and forehead and cause tension headache. If we can recognize it in its early stages we can often ease it simply by relaxing those muscles, if necessary by massaging the forehead or temple area. This is preferable to taking aspirins, which does nothing for those tense muscles but relieves pain by rendering our brain numb and insensitive to pain stimuli.

Migraine

Migraine headache is different from tension headache and is much more complex. It tends to occur in people who are perfectionists, often when they relax after intense activity. Physiologically, some blood vessels in the head (and often in the hand and other areas, too) first contract, then suddenly relax. The contraction of blood vessels in the head is responsible for the preliminary symptoms of visual or other sensory disturbance, while the dilatation of the blood vessels is responsible for the migraine's throbbing character. Disturbance in the tone of blood vessels in the stomach can lead to nausea or vomiting. The pain in the head may be so severe that the person may become totally incapacitated. A hereditary tendency, work overload, and certain foods like cheese, chocolate, yogurt, or wine may trigger an attack. Relaxation training often reduces the frequency or severity of attacks. Sometimes biofeedback training, in which the sufferer learns to raise the temperature of the hand or change the caliber of brain vessels, may be beneficial.

Backache

Prolonged bracing of trunk muscles can lead to discomfort between the shoulder blades or to lower backache. In conditions of stress and anxiety physical discomfort may become magnified, either consciously or unconsciously, and may lead to disproportionate disability. Thus a chronic domestic worry, bereavement, an unsatisfying job or the possibility of job loss, a relationship problem, or financial pressure may change lower back discomfort into intractable pain, and prolonged persistent pain may lead to profound disturbance in the person's behavior patterns. Chronic backache is a leading cause of absence from work. Early recognition, rest and relaxation, and the application of heat to relieve the spasm of contracted muscles, in addition to removing stressful situations, can help relieve the pain.

Palpitation and Chest Discomfort

Palpitation means that we are aware of our heartbeat. The resting heartbeat rate ranges between 60 and 80 beats per minute. During exercise or emotional stress the rate may rise to 150 or even 200 beats per minute and we are more likely to become aware of our heartbeat. For example, we are often aware of pounding in the chest after strenuous physical exercise. Sometimes there is a premature heartbeat, which occurs earlier than it should. This premature and usually weak contraction is followed by a longer pause and a stronger contraction. Such occurrences are often experienced as being "as if my heart turned over" or "as if my heart missed a beat." Stress, anxiety, excessive coffee or alcohol, and excessive cigarette smoking are frequently the cause, but unless and until we are aware of this possibility, palpitation can lead to unnecessary worry or investigations.

Prolonged tension in the chest muscles or a habit of breath holding can lead to chest discomfort and the fear that something may be wrong with the heart. Such worry may accentuate the tension and increase discomfort. If in doubt, go to the doctor. It is better to be safe than sorry and no doctor will mind if it turns out not to be angina (genuine heart pain) but a chest pain of another origin.

Allergies

Allergies are the body's reaction to foreign substances to which the person has become allergic. Further exposure to that substance produces antibodies in the blood which react to the offending agent. As a result several chemicals, particularly histamine and serotonin, are released and a typical allergic condition is produced. It can show in many different ways: hay fever, streaming nose, runny eyes, swollen eyelids, skin rash, asthma, itching, bleeding from the gut, or vomiting. The offending agent could be one of several things, including strawberries, chocolate, or other foodstuffs; drugs like penicillin or aspirin; dust or pollen; household chemicals like detergents; and hair spray. In fact one can become allergic to almost anything. Even if stress does not directly cause allergy it often precipitates allergic reactions in afflicted individuals. These reactions then become a source of stress, and the sufferer is locked in a vicious circle.

Colds and Coughs

Virus infections are known to cause common colds. Overcrowding and cigarette smoking are known to increase the risk but despite exposure to a virus not everyone gets a cold. So what makes one person susceptible and another resistant? Graham and co-workers from Australia studied 235 adults over a period of six months (44). The participants were divided into low-stress and high-stress groups according to the number of life events, daily hassles, and psychological states measured by the Life Events Inventory, Daily Hassles Scale, and General Health Questionnaire. The high-stress group had suffered from a significantly greater number of episodes and their symptoms lasted longer than those of the low-stress group. A number of studies have shown that stress reduces the effectiveness of our immune system. This could be the underlying mechanism relating stress and various diseases, including cancer.

Asthma

In an asthmatic attack, small bronchial tubes carrying air in and out of the lungs are narrowed because of a spasm of the muscle fibers under the influence of histamine and other chemicals released, during an allergic reaction, within the walls of the tubes. The narrowing is further aggravated by swelling of the tubes' linings, which also get covered with a sticky mucus. As a result it becomes increasingly difficult to get enough air and the affected person becomes short of breath and coughs. Breathing becomes noisy, and since bronchial tubes are narrowed further during exhalation, there is a characteristic wheezing during this phase of breathing. It can be a frightening experience which in itself can make things worse.

In susceptible individuals the attack can be precipitated by allergens, which can be one or more of many: dust, feathers, dry rot, fungus bacteria, pollens, and in some cases certain foodstuffs or drugs. The person's own cast-off dead skin cells containing house dust mites, which are collected in bedding or a mattress, are often the offending agents. Once the bronchial tubes are sensitized, other irritants, like cigarette smoke, fumes, and even steam from a hot bath, as well as psychological factors, can precipitate wheezing. In some cases exertion can bring on a wheezing attack. So, while it is not all in the mind, learning to relax, not panicking when minor wheezing starts, and using other ways of reducing stress can make asthma more manageable, in conjunction with other appropriate treatment and preventive strategies.

Angina

Angina pectoris is the Latin name for pain in the chest. It is often simply known as *angina*. It is a tight, vicelike or gripping pain in the center of the chest behind the breastbone, often radiating to the left or sometimes both arms, the neck, the throat, or the jaw. It occurs when the heart is not receiving enough oxygen for the demand at hand. The heart muscle is supplied with fresh oxygen-carrying blood by a network of small arteries known as *coronaries*. In a condition called *atherosclerosis* or *hardening of the arteries*, fatty deposits known as *plaques* are laid within the lining of the arteries. These plaques cause uneven tension in the walls of the arteries and may eventually cause cracks and bleeding inside them. The inside of the arteries becomes narrowed and irregular. When extra demands are put on the heart during exercise or following a heavy meal, exposure to cold weather, or undue emotional stress, the narrowed arteries are unable to supply extra oxygen-carrying blood. This inability leads to the typical pain of the angina, which is relieved within two or three minutes of the person's stopping all activity or calming down.

Anxiety or fear or emotional crisis releases stress hormones like epinephrine and norepinephrine, and they can increase the chances of having an anginal attack in several different ways. First, they accelerate the force and speed of the heart, thus increasing its workload. Second, they cause constriction of the blood vessels and a rise in blood pressure, and since the heart has to pump against a higher pressure, its work is increased still further. Third, they also cause constriction of the coronary arteries, narrowing further already narrowed arteries. Many cases of angina and even some cases of heart attacks have been documented through a special X-ray technique (called *angiography*) of visualizing coronary blood vessels, in which the cause is shown to be the spasm of perfectly normal coronary arteries.

Some people hyperventilate under stress. Hyperventilation is discussed in more detail in Chapter 9, "Breathing." In short, hyperventilation washes out carbon dioxide from the blood too fast, thus changing the chemical composition of the blood and making it more alkaline. Such a change in the biochemistry of the blood brings about a constriction of the coronary vessels that leads to angina. Angina itself may be frightening and therefore likely to cause further stress, thus aggravating the condition further. Drugs like nitroglycerine, which dilate blood vessels, may help to relieve an attack but they usually do nothing to cure the root cause of the condition. When angina patients are able to take vacations and force themselves away from the pressures of daily working lives, frequently their angina episodes are reduced significantly, thus pointing out its link with stress.

High Blood Pressure

Mild to moderately raised blood pressure is a common condition which affects as many as one in five adults. It can strain the heart and contribute to hardening of the arteries or atherosclerosis, the consequences of which are premature heart attacks, strokes, and other blood vessel diseases. Only in 5 to 10 percent of patients with high blood pressure is there a known cause such as kidney disease, hormone-secreting tumors, congenital malformation of certain blood vessels, or reaction to contraceptive pills. In the rest, no known cause is found. Obesity may be an associated factor in some cases but there are a huge number of thin people who also have high blood pressure (100).

Stress, excessive salt, and excessive alcohol are increasingly being recognized as contributory factors. Blood pressures are low in primitive communities where life is slow and social positions more stable. With industrialization, urbanization, and migration, social, cultural, and economic values change and people are required to make continual behavior adaptations. As people get older this process of adaptation becomes more and more stressful. This may be the reason why blood pressure rises with old age in industrialized societies and why the phenomenon is absent in primitive societies.

Certain jobs require intense alertness, as even slight mistakes can have disastrous consequences, and this requirement is often reflected in an early rise in blood pressure. For example, air traffic controllers working with high-density traffic and stockbrokers seem to have higher blood pressure than most. At the other end of the spectrum, people with boring jobs or people who lose their jobs also have high blood pressure. To quote Ogilvie, "Hypertension is a new disease and a stress disease, the price a millionaire pays for his directorship and a clerk for his failure" (95). A number of studies have now shown that regular practice of relaxation and learning to manage stress effectively can lead to a significant reduction in high blood pressure (101). This observation alone suggests that stress must be an important contributing causal factor.

Heart Attacks

High blood pressure, a high level of cholesterol fat in the blood, and cigarette smoking are considered major risk factors for coronary heart disease, but in half the patients who suffer from heart attacks none of these factors are present (100). Even when minor or less important risk factors like obesity, diabetes, and lack of physical activity are taken into consideration, there is still a large number of patients for whom the cause of heart attack remains unknown.

When blood cells clump together to produce a clot called a *thrombus*, the blood supply through that part of the coronary network is completely cut off. This is what happens during a heart attack. Cigarette smoking, as well as stress hormones, is known to increase the stickiness of blood cells and thus the tendency to form the clot. The chest pain which ensues is similar to angina but occurs at rest and lasts much longer. The part of the heart muscle supplied by the blocked section dies and is eventually replaced by a scar.

There are a number of other reasons why it is doubtful that known risk factors give the full story. When patients with all three major risk factors discussed above were followed for ten years, only 13 percent succumbed to heart attacks; the rest remained apparently well. So what precipitates a heart attack? The importance of diet is not denied but it has to be said that the consumption of saturated fat like lard, suet, butter, cream, cheese, and fatty meat has remained almost unchanged and may even have gone down in the last sixty years, while the number of coronary heart attacks has increased dramatically during that time. Freezing has largely replaced salt in the preservation of meat, fruit, and vegetables yet high blood pressure and heart attacks seem to be more common. Even though a husband and wife eat the same food, the husband is three times more likely to have a heart attack.

There are many reasons why stress may be another important contributing factor. In population surveys in both the United States and the United Kingdom people have voted stress to be the number one causative factor for both heart attacks and high blood pressure. What is the basis of such folk wisdom? Bereavement for the conjugal partner is probably the most stressful life event known to us. The fact that stress can kill through the heart is not simply folklore but has been shown in a number of studies; grievers seem to be at a much greater risk of heart attack than nongrievers.

Risk factors are important, but what are their underlying causes? Diet is responsible for only a part of the total presence of cholesterol fat in the blood, the rest being manufactured within the body (138). It has been shown to rise in medical students during the last months of preparation for final examinations, in accountants during intense activity before tax deadlines, in cadets admitted to the U.S. Air Force Academy during the initial and most stressful weeks, and in underwater-demolition-team trainees when under the stress of learning a new and dangerous skill. A stress-prone personality, particularly one showing a Type A behavior pattern, is considered another risk factor. We have already discussed this in Chapter 3.

In one study my colleagues and I (103) identified 192 men and women, through a screening program in one industry, who were at higher than normal risk of developing heart disease because of the presence of two of the three risk factors: (1) mildly raised blood pressure not considered high enough for drug therapy; (2) mildly elevated blood cholesterol, for which there was no other treatment than dietary advice; and (3) smoking of ten or more cigarettes a day. We randomized our subjects into control and treatment groups. Both groups were given the advice to stop smoking, dietary advice to reduce their intake of saturated fat and salt, and appropriate information on high blood pressure. The treatment group received, in addition, training in mental and physical relaxation and ways of reducing stress. The blood pressure of this group was significantly lower at each of the three examinations we carried out, after eight weeks, eight months, and four years. Over the four years there were six cases of coronary heart disease in the control group, including one fatal attack, while in the treatment group there was only one abnormality of the electrical tracing of the heart indicating possible coronary heart disease. This observation on its own does not prove the stress hypothesis but strongly suggests that it may be correct. I later trained other doctors who in turn treated their own high-blood-pressure patients. One year later we observed five cases of coronary heart disease in the control group compared with one complication in the treatment group (102). The same results twice are unlikely to be due to chance alone. The added bonus was improved quality of life with this therapy, contrary to the results of many drug treatments which give rise to undesirable side effects (101).

Chronic Fatigue

The feeling of being tired all the time is probably the commonest symptom of stress. Fatigue is a feeling of having insufficient energy to carry on and a strong desire to stop, rest, or sleep. It is a weariness that comes from either physical or mental exertion. Fatigue is described in the dictionary as a feeling of tiredness, exhaustion, weariness, of being weak, haggard, lethargic, languid, listless, bushed, drowsy, sleepy, sluggish, pooped out, or worn out. Actually fatigue is a subjective feeling and has several predictable behavioral and physical effects. Dr. Holly Atkinson (2) states:

> Aside from feeling weary, tired persons are unable to deal effectively with complex problems and tend to be unreasonable, often about trivialities. The ability to deliberate and to reach judgment is impaired, decisions made late

at night may appear unsound the next day. The worker after a long hard day is unable to perform adequately his or her duties as a head of a household; the example of the tired business person who becomes the proverbial tyrant of the circle is well known.

Fatigue may be associated with the physical sensations of headache, dizziness, nausea, and tremulousness. Dr. Atkinson suggests that we look at fatigue as a signal of energy imbalance; too much energy is being expended and not enough energy is being boosted or conserved. Stress, whether physical, mental, or emotional, drains us of energy, as do stress-associated behaviors like smoking, alcohol use, or drug use, while good nutrition, exercise, sleep, pleasure, and achieving mastery over situations boost our energy to deal with the problems and demands of life. Fatigue disturbs our moods, our concentration, our perceptions, our capacity to work and play, and our capacity to love. It takes the sparkle out of life.

Unfortunately fatigue is not taken seriously. The usual response of doctors to the complaint of fatigue is to order a battery of tests and to report that all the test results are normal, meaning that there is nothing physically wrong or that it is all in the mind. Such statements do severe injustice to the patient, who is made to believe either that the fatigue is a figment of the imagination or that its basis is all psychological and therefore not important. Chronic fatigue deserves due attention in the promotion of health.

Anxiety State

When exposed to a threatening situation like going for a job interview, going to the dentist or doctor, or taking an important examination, it is normal to feel anxious. It is part of the stress response, which also makes us tense and vigilant as we wait for new information, wait to make a decision and then probably to act. In that state we may be uncertain at one stage, hopeful at another, and hopeless and despairing at another. We may tremble, our hands may feel cold and clammy, and there may be feelings of fluttering in the chest, a sinking feeling in the stomach, or an increase in the breathing rate. These may not be abnormal if we recover soon. In some people the threshold for anxiety is low, and quite trivial events can be enough to cause a wave of anxiety and anticipation of imminent catastrophe. Simple things like the breakdown of a washing machine or news of an accident on TV may be perceived as a major crisis. Sometimes the worry is justified, for instance, if there are family or financial problems or the threat of job loss is looming in the background. However, given time we make adjustments to all such situations.

In the anxiety state, the fear is so severe, persistent, and pervasive that it colors every thought during every waking moment. There is an overwhelming sense of foreboding that something terrible is about to happen. The mind is full of problems on waking up, and when one goes to bed they are still unresolved. As anxiety deepens, stress becomes more intense until the individual is reacting to almost everything in life. A slight noise will make him jump out of his skin, and in severe cases he is living with sheer terror. Not being able to define the problem makes the feeling of dread even worse. The affected person becomes snappish and irritable, his mind may be unable to pay attention to work, and he may feel a sense of unreality about himself. More women complain about anxiety than men. Normal stress reactions are exaggerated and are described in the following kinds of ways: "My heart felt it was going to stop"; "I have aches and pains all over"; "I feel tired all the time"; "There is a tight band round my head"; "I just can't get enough breath"; "Sex doesn't interest me"; "I have completely gone off my food"; "It takes hours before I can fall asleep and then I wake up drenched in cold sweats after a nightmare"; or "I know my fears are irrational but I can't get rid of them."

Many anxiety sufferers are subject to panic attacks, which are acute episodes of anxiety associated with physical symptoms like palpitation, sweating, and even fainting. On hearing stressful news, like of the death of a close friend, such a person may actually collapse and lose consciousness. The anxious person has a tendency to arouse anxiety in others, who either seek to avoid him or tell him to pull himself together. Either reaction will increase the isolation of the anxious person and the feeling that no one understands him.

Phobias

A phobia is an irrational fear which is completely out of proportion to the particular situation. A common one is agoraphobia, or fear of open space. The person is afraid to go to public places or crowded shops. Claustrophobia is fear of darkness or closed spaces. Such phobias are a menace to daily living. A phobia may come out of the blue, but for many people it is the aftermath of a period of great stress which may have been caused by a bereavement, an illness, or other trauma. A fighter pilot may become agoraphobic after receiving a bombing injury. In a sense it is a delayed reaction to critical events. Sometimes people have specific phobias in which there is unreasonable fear of specific things like dogs, cats, snakes, spiders, or birds. For such people living in the country is a nightmare. People afraid of elevators climb endless stairs. Those who know their handicap are under a lot of stress. The usual treatment is called *desensitization*, in which the patient is first taught relaxation and then is gradually exposed to the situations which cause fear. Imaginary situations are used at first and later real ones. Such people can be helped by local self-help groups.

Depression

Loss of someone or something significant in one's life, as in bereavement, loss of a job, divorce, or the surgical removal of the womb, can lead to a feeling of despair and depression. This feeling state is quite natural, and usually, in time, it gradually lifts and the person is able to cope with life once more. If, on the other hand, such a feeling pervades the person's whole life, it becomes an abnormal reaction. Such depression may appear out of the blue, when it is known as *endogenous* or *internally generated depression*. However, it is now thought that even these depressive states are triggered by stressful events (40).

Postnatal Depression

When depression develops after the birth of a baby it is called *postnatal depression*. This is different from the usual "baby blues," a brief weepy period which frequently occurs three to four days after the birth; it is more insidious and sets in some weeks after the birth. The cause is not well understood but it is thought that the physical and emotional stress of giving birth to and looking after the baby, with the associated loss of freedom and perhaps also of a career, may precipitate depression in a woman who is predisposed to such a reaction to stress.

Depressive Illness

An overwhelming stress can deplete the brain of epinephrine and other, related chemicals, resulting in a depressive illness. The most pervading symptoms of depressive illness are the feeling of emptiness, lack of interest, and loss of energy. The person is unable to enjoy life or work. Everything looks bleak, food is tasteless, flowers are odorless, and scenery is colorless. It is hard to get moving. It may be difficult to move from a chair or to get out of bed; the body feels physically heavy and may appear slumped; movements get slower and it takes longer and longer to complete normal tasks; or the person just feels slowed down. Mental agility is lost and the person procrastinates longer and longer rather than make decisions. As a result he may lose his job or housework may be neglected. He feels so hopeless that the belief in life, the belief in goodness, and the belief in hope itself get lost. Friends and relatives who try to help are rejected, as are previous interests and hobbies.

There is no feeling. A depressed person can look at his own child and feel no tenderness. If someone provokes him, he feels indifferent instead of angry. No efforts are made to maintain personal hygiene or appearance. The melody and harmony of music he loves lose their appeal. The deepening of depression involves a gradual abdication of responsibility. The affected person is unable to concentrate and memory becomes poor. In short, life feels overwhelmingly lifeless, as if an all-enveloping black cloud descends and permeates everything that exists, coloring everything black and gray. Occasionally depression is accompanied by bouts of irritability or agitation, especially in the elderly. The person may feel that life is not worth living and may attempt suicide. Sometimes there is a feeling of self-pity and unfairness which becomes self-perpetuating and stops the person from taking positive action. Humor is avoided at all costs. There may be physical symptoms like headache, backache, and shooting pains. If a painful condition already existed before the depressive illness, the pain becomes worse. The person may imagine he has an incurable cancer or some other dreadful disease.

Sleep patterns may be profoundly affected. It may be difficult to fall asleep or the person may wake up very early feeling dreadfully depressed. Some young patients may oversleep. The depressed person often loses his appetite and loses weight; often there is a loss of libido or sexual drive. Some drink heavily and this only makes things worse. Occasionally both anxiety state and depressive illness are combined.

The treatment of depression requires a great deal of understanding by health care providers as well as friends and relatives, in addition to antidepressant drugs to correct a biochemical imbalance in the brain.

Irritable Bowel Syndrome

Often known as *irritable colon* or *spastic colon*, this is a condition in which the afflicted person gets colicky lower abdominal pain, diarrhea alternating with constipation, frequency of stools with a feeling that the bowel has not completely emptied, and occasionally distension or a bloated feeling. In some, constipation is the predominant symptom. Stress may not be very important in this category of afflicted individuals; lack of fiber in the diet may be more relevant. In others, diarrhea, distension, and pain, due to spasms of the bowel walls, are the predominant feature, and in these cases stress may be more relevant. Treatment should deal with the sources of stress and should include an increase in dietary fibers with additional fresh fruit, vegetables, and wholemeal bread, as well as drugs to relieve colonic spasm. In other similar but less common conditions known as *ulcerative colitis* and *Crohn's disease*, the bowel becomes ulcerated and stools often contain blood and mucus. Both are chronic conditions with periods of exacerbation and remission. Stress is often an exacerbating factor. Treatment involves hospital supervision; drugs, including steroids; and stress reduction.

Peptic Ulcer

This is a condition in which there is a breach in the lining of the stomach (gastric ulcer) or the upper part of the bowel (duodenal ulcer). Occasionally erosion occurs in the lower part of the gullet or food pipe (esophageal ulcer). The most obvious symptom is pain. The most common is the duodenal ulcer, in which the pain typically occurs when the stomach is empty, thus often waking the person up in the middle of the night. Eating or drinking milk often stops the pain. People with gastric ulcer, on the other hand, often find their pain becomes worse after eating. Sometimes people have typical pain but no ulcer is detected by a special barium-meal X ray or by a fiber-optic endoscopy in which a flexible tube is passed into the stomach through the food pipe and the doctor views the lining of the stomach and the duodenum directly.

The secretion of acid in the stomach plays a crucial role in the causation of peptic ulcer and the typical pain. Normally the stomach protects itself against the burning effect of the acid by secreting a layer of mucus. It is believed that stress and sometimes certain anti-inflammatory drugs used for arthritis, painkillers, and cigarette smoking can cause or aggravate the condition by causing more acid and less mucus to be secreted. Certain occupations—such as air traffic control—are considered more stressful and thus more liable to lead to ulcers. Food neutralizes the acid and thus relieves the pain. If people go without food for many hours, the acid accumulates and may begin to damage the lining of the stomach, especially if the mucus coating is defective. A person suffering from peptic ulcers can help himself by eating small meals frequently, and by avoiding alcohol, spicy and fried food, smoking, stressful situations, and painkillers like aspirin and other anti-inflammatory drugs. It should be remembered that aspirin is sold in many guises—acetyl salicylic acid, salicylic acid, sodium salicylate, and so on. Doctors usually prescribe antacids in the form of liquid or tablets. There is a tendency for the condition to return unless efforts are made to change the conditions which caused the ulcer in the first place.

Premenstrual Syndrome

A woman who is subject to premenstrual syndrome (PMS) feels anxious, unduly sensitive, and tense a few days before her period. Stress is often a contributing factor, and when suffering from PMS she is not likely to cope with day-to-day stress as well as she does at other times of the month. Symptoms may be physical, like fatigue; breast tenderness; water retention; bloating of the stomach; swelling of the ankles, feet, or fingers; and joint pains. There may be headaches, migraines, backaches, cold sores, or worsening of acne spots. Mentally she may be anxious, tense, depressed, irritable, weepy, confused, and often forgetful. Relaxation and counseling are helpful. Sometimes diuretics, tranquilizers, or hormone treatments are prescribed by the doctor, depending on the predominant symptoms.

Diabetes Mellitus

Acute symptoms of diabetes, like intense thirst and excessive urine flow, may first appear after an accident, illness, or emotional crisis or may be discovered for the first time during a pregnancy or after a heart attack. It may be that stress unmasks the latent condition rather than causes diabetes in a previously undiagnosed person.

If someone is already under treatment for diabetes, physical or emotional stress may cause a worsening of blood sugar control. Such worsening is well known after an infection, a heart attack, or an accident and is less common after an emotional crisis. However, like any chronic condition whose regimen requires severe personal discipline, diabetes itself can cause considerable stress, and adolescents and children are particularly likely to rebel against the dietary restrictions and the harshness of treatment regimen.

EFFECTS OF WORK STRESS

In many ways the effect of work stress is no different from that of any other stress. Therefore the warning signs, as well as the stress-related illnesses already discussed, apply to work stress as well. However there are certain syndrome or symptom complexes which are specific to work stress, and these are described below.

Workaholism

People get addicted not only to alcohol and smoking but to anything that becomes so central that life seems impossible without it. For many, the workplace, the organization they work for, and the job they do are central focuses in their lives. Work itself may also be very addictive. Addiction serves to numb us so that we are out of touch with ourselves and our feelings, a state in which we are neither dead nor fully alive but like a zombie, although fully occupied. Ann Wilson Schaef and Diane Fassel (118) suggest that society and corporations foster this addiction because if we are dead we are not much good for work and if we are fully alive we will revolt against many things. Society prefers to look the other way, toward racism, polluted environments, the nuclear threat, the arms race, unsafe water, carcinogenic foods, or poverty. The promises held out by organizations or companies, written or unwritten, effectively removed our attention from the acute and sometimes appalling problems of the present and fix it on a rosy picture of the future when the promissory note will bear fruit and the dream of money, power, or influence in the form of a pay raise, bonuses, or a higher position leading to higher social status will all be ours for the taking. This picture of the good life, reinforced by popular culture, becomes so seductive that we are prepared to abide by rigid rules and regulations, to forget our family and friends, to work our fingers to the bone, and to remain constantly alert, so that we do not say or do things that might bring about our fall from grace in the company.

There is nothing wrong with being dedicated to our work or being loyal to our employer. It is only when this dedication becomes a preoccupation, a substitute for our personal life, that it becomes a fix. As with any addiction, the company's commission, bonuses, or pension scheme becomes the sole controlling factor in the lives of employees, to the point that they sometimes cross the boundary of morality: a salesman will sell you something which he knows is not appropriate for your needs, or a researcher will produce falsified results.

It is not only permissible but even fashionable to say, "I am a workaholic and I love it." This would not be said so proudly about addiction to alcohol or marijuana, and yet workaholism can be as destructive to our health as any other addiction. It ruins relationships both at home and at work. Divorce and separation are common among those who have reached the top by their "hard work." They often drop dead without receiving medical attention, because they are under tremendous stress but utterly deny it. It may be that what they are addicted to is not their work but the adrenaline high that accompanies it. Many workaholics describe the surge of energy they get while at work, which they identify as a thrilling experience, one of excitement or being totally alive. No wonder they feel bored when they are on vacation, for it is like sending an alcoholic to a water spa and expecting him to enjoy it.

For most of us, time between projects is time to recuperate, to feel a sense of accomplishment, and to savor the achievement. But not so for workaholics. They loathe these quiet periods of low-key work. They are deprived of their adrenaline. If they are not striving to control their environment, they feel they are being controlled by it, a situation which they detest. Adrenaline allows us to perform extraordinary tasks during a crisis but our body is not built to withstand a constant surge of adrenaline. Modern corporate life tricks us into believing that there is a constant crisis.

Burnout

One of the most common and often unrecognized syndromes of job stress is burnout. Like a disease, it progresses slowly and goes through recognizable stages. Dr. Robert Veninga and Dr. James Spradly describe five stages (139).

Stage of Job Contentment. The individual is happy with the job he does. He puts in more and more energy, but if it is not replenished in good time or adequately, the second stage is gradually reached.

Stage of Fuel Shortage. The person begins to feel tired, there is a lack of energy, and sleep becomes disturbed. He begins to complain of not being able to do as many things as he once did; creativity is at a low; there is a tendency to avoid making decisions and toward increased cynicism.

Stage of Chronic Symptoms. He begins to feel exhausted and may feel physically ill. There are vague symptoms like bodyache, nausea, tension headaches, or back pain. There is a tendency to wake up in the morning feeling tired. A once calm, easygoing person becomes chronically angry or always on the verge of losing his temper.

Stage of Crisis. Symptoms become critical. Periods when the person's thoughts are not riveted on the job are increasingly rare. The mind is constantly preoccupied with work problems, even when the person is watching television or having family dinner. At times there is an overwhelming urge to escape from it all—the job, the family, and the whole way of life.

Stage of Final Breakdown. Finally, the person feels unable to continue. Some drown themselves in alcohol and drugs. Others have a mental or physical breakdown in the form of depression or a heart attack. There is serious deterioration in the functioning of one or more organs of the body.

Take a good look at yourself, your feelings and symptoms, and your job. If you are experiencing the early warning signs of fuel shortage, do something before you reach the state of chronic symptoms. If you are already experiencing symptoms, there is no time to waste before you take appropriate steps. If you are already in the crisis stage, drop everything and take immediate action to prevent a breakdown.

II

How to Cope with Stress

9

Breathing

Breathing is essential to life. Life begins with a person's first breath and ends with the last. Breathing is automatic and usually involuntary, being controlled, like all other internal functions, by the autonomic or involuntary nervous system, and as we are not aware of all internal functions, we are not normally aware of breathing. The brain filters out many of the events that are happening constantly in order to focus on the more important things at hand. Things which are important for immediate survival are given top priority. Many people, if not most, breathe shallowly and haphazardly, going against the natural rhythmic movements of the respiratory system. Thus, despite the fact that breathing is one of the most vital functions of the body, it is often done improperly and is little understood. However, breathing is also unique in that it can be controlled by an act of will. Since we breathe between 16,000 and 20,000 times a day, breathing can be a very powerful tool in gaining some degree of control over our autonomic functions. Recent research, particularly biofeedback research, has shown that several internal functions previously thought to be out of the mental realm can, in fact, be brought under our own control. In order to exert a certain degree of control over the functioning of our body and mind it is important to understand the process of breathing.

BREATHING ACCORDING TO YOGA AND ITS SCIENTIFIC MEANING

Yoga masters spend years learning the intricate aspects of breathing (110). They have discovered that besides the body and the mind there are other levels of existence; the one which links the body and the mind is the level of functioning and the one that lies beyond the mind or thoughts is a consciousness or the level of heightened and broadened awareness. The level of existence that links the body with the mind has something to do with the energy concept. In fact we cannot study the body without becoming aware that it functions because of energy.

But what is energy? Einstein gave the formula $E = mc^2$, where E = energy and m = matter. The formula thus implies not only that matter and energy bear a definite relationship to each other, but also that they are interconvertible. The most dramatic example of matter being converted into energy is the atomic explosion. In Sanskrit, India's most ancient language, the level of functioning that involves energy is called *prana*, which literally means "life force." Some 3,000 years ago, yogis with highly developed extrasensory perception pronounced that "life is in the breath," and by breath they meant more than just the lungs, the blood circulation, and the gaseous exchange which takes place between inspired air and blood circulating in the lungs. Even now, when someone gets a creative insight into something we call it an inspiration. When we hear great and wise people talking we get inspired or we call these talks inspired talks. The more *prana* or life force we have, the greater our physical energy and mental alertness and awareness. The person who radiates vitality and energy and who has a kind of magnetic personality has more abundance of life force.

But what is this *prana*, or life force? Here we return to breath, because breath is considered the vehicle for *prana*.

When someone dies, and the life force has left, we say he has expired because that life energy has left with the last breath. Thus, through the language we use, we convey an intuitive recognition of the relationship between breath and vital energy, its indispensability for life and for creativity. We all experience, from time to time, a great deal of vitality and clarity of mind, while at other times we experience a sense of having no mental energy. In addition to breath, we also derive energy from food, water, and sunshine.

The flow of breath is constantly helping the process that underlies and sustains the physical body. It creates and sustains the tissues of the body. If some part is poorly supplied with this energy it will become sick. If breath influences both the body and the mind, not only are physical, mental, and emotional states reflected in the pattern of breath but through breathing we can also influence our physical, psychological, and spiritual well-being.

Yoga philosophy does not pay much attention to the individual and his uniqueness. It does not believe in the *I*. In fact, there is a positive longing to unite with the universe. Most of us believe ourselves to be genetically unique individuals, different from anyone and everyone, and yet this is nothing but an illusion according to Dr. Larry Dossey (25). The basic component of all genes is the protein DNA, and the life span of any single DNA is short-lived, no more than a few months. Even though the pattern remains the same, the protein stuff of which the genes are made is constantly changing. The thousands of individual carbon, hydrogen, oxygen, and other atoms that comprise it are in constant exchange with the world outside. The modern technique of using radioisotopes that allow us to trace the chemicals that enter and leave the body demonstrates that 98 percent of the atoms of the entire body are replaced every year. Each structure of the body has its own rate of re-formation: the lining of the stomach renews itself in one week, the skin is entirely replaced in a month, and the liver is regenerated within six weeks. Some tissues are relatively slow to turn over, for example, the supporting tissue of the body called *collagen*. The bone, on the other hand, is specially dynamic. Our bodies are thus constantly dissolving and renewing themselves. We all know that in the next five years we will have completely renewed our hair and our nails, but did you know that in five years' time not a single atom of your present body will be here and that five years ago you didn't exist? This is the eerie quality of human life, says Dossey, the author of *Space, Time and Medicine*. In the constant dissolution of our genetic selves we retain a sense of an unchanging physical *I*. Our dissolution is a silent flow occurring outside our awareness.

There is a constant flow of new parts from the earth and everything we see on the earth. In fact the boundary extends beyond the earth itself. It is known that certain elements in the body, such as the phosphorus in our bones, were formed at an earlier stage in the evolution of our galaxy. Like many elements in the earth's crust, it was cycled through a lifetime of several stars before appearing on the earth and finding its way through to our bodies. The carbon atom that is part of me now will become part of the earth and may become part of someone or something else later. There is a constant dynamic biodance, a persistent equilibrium, an endless exchange of elements between living things and the earth. The idea that we shall return to where we came from makes some sense, except that we do not wait until death. We are constantly returning to the earth while we are alive! We seem to be part of a basic oneness with the universe. Breathing provides a vital link in this equilibrium. Even with our simple knowledge of human physiology we know that the oxygen we breathe is very important in the metabolic process. Without it, we cannot burn energy, the continuous supply of which is necessary to continue functioning. Without it, the nourishment we take cannot be utilized to repair and regenerate our body. Plants absorb the carbon dioxide we breathe out and, using the process of photosynthesis in the presence of sunlight, release oxygen into the atmosphere. But breathing is more than that.

Did you know that the average breath you breathe contains about 10 sextillion atoms, a number which can be written in modern notation as 10^{22}? Since the entire atmosphere of the earth is voluminous enough to contain 10^{22} breaths, we can say that every time you inhale, you are, on average, drawing one atom from each of these breaths, and that every time you exhale, you are, on average, sending one atom to each of these breaths in the sky, and so is every one else. This exchange is repeated some 16,000 to 20,000 times a day by some 6 billion people living on this planet. It has been calculated that each breath you breathe must contain a quadrillion, or 10^{15}, atoms breathed by the rest of humankind within the last few weeks and more than a million atoms breathed personally, at some time, by each and every person on earth.

Thus without exception we are all partners in this bio-dance. There is no question about the fact that the mind affects the body but it also seems certain that everyone affects everyone else and breathing seems to be the medium. That is why we sometimes say, "The atmosphere was congenial," or "The air was rather tense." The only way to find peace and harmony for ourselves and with everyone and everything that exists in this universe is through love.

We have established through mathematical science that all breathing creatures share the same oxygen molecules, creating a low-frequency chain of chemical contacts between all living creatures. We even share these atoms and molecules with plants which give us the oxygen we need and assimilate the carbon dioxide we release. The question is: What is the significance of this contact at the level of human experience? We know that since ancient times there have been people, the so-called mystics, who claimed to have a direct sense of contact with others, an experience of unity with all human beings at all times. Could they possibly be right? Is it just a question of paying attention?

BREATHING AND EMOTION

Our breathing pattern reflects our state of mind and emotions. For example, an anxious person tends to breathe rapidly and often, using only the upper part of the chest; a depressed person tends to sigh; a person who gets hysterical tends to overbreathe, the condition often known as *hyperventilation;* a child during a temper tantrum holds his breath until he is blue in the face. The anxious person talks at the end of an inhalation in a high-tone voice. The depressed person talks at the end of an exhalation in a low-toned voice. In fact, what is going on in the totality of a person can be judged by the pattern of his breathing. This information is available all the time, the information that reflects the essence of our physical and mental state, but we are almost completely unaware of it. The most fascinating story is being told but we do not seem to be comprehending it; a revealing kind of information is being released but we are not receiving it.

COSMIC BREATHING

Astronomers of modern times, using the most sophisticated instruments, have found that the distances between the galaxies are increasing. Through their calculations, they have concluded that the galaxies and planets are pulling apart from each other, that the whole universe is expanding or swelling, so to speak. The most coherent theory at present is that all this movement has resulted from a sort of explosion from a center. This is known as the *Big Bang Theory*, according to which the universe is expanding and after a certain point will again begin to contract and all the planets, solar systems, and galaxies will be pulled back together to a point from which the universe will all expand again. The process sounds a familiar one, that of expansion and contraction, similar to inhalation and exhalation, but this time involving not an individual human being but the cosmos, as if in cosmic breathing.

CELLULAR RESPIRATION

All organisms, human, plant, or animal, are composed of many tiny individual units called *cells*. These cells are organized into specific tissues or organs which together form the physical body. The life and functioning of these cells depend on a continuous source of energy. The food we eat has to be converted into a form which can be used by the cells. The nourishment we take is absorbed into the bloodstream and eventually supplied to individual cells. To produce energy, it must combine with oxygen in a process known as *oxidation*. This process takes place within subunits of each cell, called *mitochondria*, which contain the enzyme cytochrome oxidase. This enzyme takes the energy released by the oxidation of food and transfers it to an energy storage molecule called *adenosine triphosphate*, or ATP, which releases it when the body needs it.

THE RESPIRATORY SYSTEM

Before oxygen can reach the cells it has to travel through the lungs and the blood circulation. The air is inhaled through the nose and travels down the windpipe, known as the *trachea*. The trachea divides into two smaller tubes, one supplying each lung. These tubes, known as *bronchi*, branch off, getting smaller and smaller until they become microscopic in size. After about fifteen generations of branching they terminate in tiny tubes called *bronchioles*, each of which ends in a series of tiny air sacs with very thin walls called *alveoli*. Surrounding the alveoli is a network of tiny blood vessels known as *capillaries*. The walls of these capillaries are so thin that gas can

easily flow through them and the inside is so narrow that blood
cells literally have to squeeze through them.

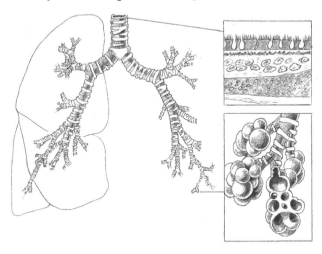

Gaseous exchange takes place between the air in the alveoli and the blood in the capillaries. Ideally there should be
a match between the amount of blood flowing through the
capillaries and the oxygen brought to the alveoli by breathing.
However, the physiology of the lungs shows that blood is not
evenly distributed throughout the entire lung. Because of grav-
ity dependence, there is more blood in the lower part of the
lung than in the upper, when one is in the upright position.
Conversely, there is more ventilation and therefore more oxygen in the upper part of the lung. Thus we have a situation
which the physiologists call *ventilation-perfusion mismatch*.
More serious inefficiencies occur if the alveoli are injured by
smoking. Most people have about 3 million alveoli in their
lungs. Slow destruction of alveoli continues for years, and it
is only when their numbers are drastically reduced that the
person may feel "short of breath."

Oxygen, once in the bloodstream, gets bound to hemoglobin molecules within the red blood cells. Hemoglobin also

picks up carbon dioxide, the waste product from the cells, and carries it to the lungs. As it takes up oxygen, it releases carbon dioxide, which diffuses into the alveoli and is then exhaled. Normally oxygen and carbon dioxide are the only molecules of gas which bind to the hemoglobin molecule. However, there is one exception. Carbon monoxide, which appears in high concentration in cigarette smoke and exhaust fumes, has an affinity for hemoglobin which is 240 times that for oxygen. If present, carbon monoxide will replace oxygen, thus decreasing the oxygen-carrying capacity of the blood. Smokers have 10 to 20 percent of their hemoglobin constantly tied up in this way.

TYPES OF BREATHING

To ensure that we will get an adequate supply of oxygen it is helpful to understand how we actually breathe. There are two main types of breathing: costal (meaning "of the ribs") or chest breathing, and diaphragmatic or abdominal breathing. Only when we take a maximum breath is a third variety used, known as clavicular breathing.

Costal or Chest Breathing

This type of breathing is characterized by an outward, upward movement of the chest wall. In chest breathing the expansion is centered at the midpoint and consequently it aerates the middle part of the lung most. Since the lower part of the lung is most abundantly perfused with blood, we have that ventilation-perfusion mismatch described earlier. Thus during resting periods chest breathing is less efficient. Chest breathing also requires more work to be done in lifting the rib cage; thus the body has to work harder to accomplish the same blood-gas mixing than with diaphragmatic breathing, and the greater the work, the greater the amount of oxygen needed, so that more frequent breaths results. Chest breathing is useful during vigorous exercise but it is quite inappropriate for ordinary, everyday activity. Since it is part and parcel of the fight-or-flight response it occurs when the individual is aroused by external or internal challenges or danger. As a result, chest breathing is likely to be associated with other symptoms of arousal, like tension and anxiety. Since there is a reciprocal relationship between breathing and the mind, chest breathing, if continued during rest periods, will lead to tension and anxiety, thus creating a vicious circle. With chest breathing the breath is likely to be shallow, jerky, and unsteady, resulting in unsteadiness of the mind and emotions. Until chest breathing is replaced by deep, even, and steady diaphragmatic breathing, all efforts to relax the body, nerves, and mind will be ineffective.

Abdominal or Diaphragmatic Breathing

The principal muscle involved in abdominal breathing is the diaphragm, a strong dome-shaped sheet of muscle that separates the chest cavity from the abdomen. When we breathe in, the diaphragm contracts and pushes downward, causing the abdominal muscles to relax and rise. In this position, the lungs expand, creating a partial vacuum which allows air to be drawn in. When we breathe out, the diaphragm relaxes, and the abdominal muscles contract and expel air containing carbon dioxide.

Of the two major types of breathing, diaphragmatic breathing is the most efficient because greater expansion and ventilation occurs in the lower part of the lung, where the blood perfusion is greatest. In children and infants the diaphragm is the sole muscle of respiration, so if you watch an infant breathing you should get a good idea of what diaphragmatic breathing is like. As the diaphragm contracts it pushes the abdominal organs downward and forward, and this rhythmical massage gently compresses the organs and improves circulation. Diaphragmatic breathing in conjunction with physical and mental relaxation has been found to reduce high blood pressure and anxiety significantly.

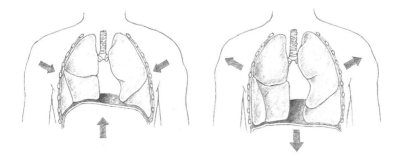

When we are calm and composed our breathing is diaphragmatic, and since there is a reciprocal relationship between breathing and the mind, practicing diaphragmatic breathing leads to mental relaxation. It is the most important tool available for stress management. It promotes a natural, even movement of breath which both strengthens the nervous system and relaxes the body. It is the most efficient method of breathing, using minimum effort for maximum oxygen. Up and down movements of the diaphragm massages the abdominal organs, improving their circulation.

The following are the main benefits:

- Providing the body with sufficient oxygen
- Expelling carbon dioxide adequately
- Relaxing the body and the mind
- Improving circulation to the abdominal organs

Clavicular Breathing

Clavicular breathing is significant only when maximum air is needed. The name is derived from the two clavicles, or collar bones, which are pulled up slightly at the end of maximum inhalation, expanding the very top of the lungs. It comes into play when the body's need for oxygen is very great. This type of breathing can be seen in patients with asthma or chronic bronchitis.

Breathing and the Brain

The inside of the nose is covered by a spongy lining rich in erectile tissue, which is involved in a continuous process of swelling and shrinking. As it gradually swells in one nostril it simultaneously shrinks in the other. The cycle is reversed approximately every one hour and forty-five minutes to two hours. As one nostril becomes relatively obstructed the airflow gradually shifts to the other side. Thus there is a right or left dominance of the airflow. Research has shown that when the air is flowing predominantly through the right nostril, we are likely to be active and aggressive, alert and oriented toward the external world—a pattern typical of left-brain predominance. When the air is flowing predominantly through the left nostril, we are more likely to be quiet, in a receptive psychological mood, intuitive, and more oriented toward the inner world—a pattern typical of right-brain predominance. Right-left nostril breathing not only reflects different psychological states but also physiological states. It is thought that airflow through the right nostril gears the internal organs to more active processes, like the digestion of food. It is said that students of Swara Yoga, a branch of Yoga particularly involved in the study of breathing, eat when the right nostril is open; they drink when the left nostril is open because drinking is a more passive kind of intake. The breath is attuned properly before undertaking a specific activity in order to maintain harmony between the mind and the body.

A type of yogic breathing known as *alternate-nostril breathing* is specially designed to restore balance between right- and left-brain functioning. Normally, in a modern society, we are attuned to the logical, rational, calculating, active left brain to such an extent that sometimes it becomes difficult to switch off when relaxation or artistic, creative, intuitive activity is preferred. In alternate-nostril breathing the flow of air is deliberately changed from one nostril to the other through blocking alternate nostrils. This has a very calming effect on the mind and helps restore sleep to those who suffer from insomnia. It should not, however, be tried until diaphragmatic breathing has been mastered. Full instructions for both diaphragmatic and alternate nostril breathing are given later in this chapter.

ABNORMAL BREATHING PATTERNS

Hyperventilation

During stress or arousal, breathing becomes faster, and even if diaphragmatic breathing was predominant until then, it now changes to chest breathing, which is more likely to meet the anticipated needs for increased oxygen. If the anticipated event results in physical activity, the body will discharge its accumulated energy, and relaxation, with its diaphragmatic breathing pattern, will be restored. If this does not happen, chest breathing may continue. As mentioned earlier, chest breathing leads to tension and anxiety, a greater amount of work and therefore faster breathing. If the perceived threat or demands continue, hyperventilation may become a habitual mode of breathing.

During rapid breathing a greater than average amount of carbon dioxide is washed out of the system. A certain amount of carbon dioxide is necessary for healthy functioning of the body. Lowering of the carbon dioxide level in the blood leads to constriction of the blood vessels in many vital organs, resulting in many diverse and often serious symptoms. For example, constriction of blood vessels in the brain may make us feel dizzy or light-headed and in extreme cases may lead to loss of consciousness. A similar process in the blood vessels of the heart may lead to chest pain, which may be indistinguishable from angina. Reduction in the level of carbon dioxide in the blood makes blood more alkaline and makes the nerves more irritable, a reaction felt as widespread tingling or pins and needles and sometimes as spasms in the muscles, giving rise to clawlike hands, pulling of the mouth, and, in severe cases, generalized convulsions.

These hyperventilators, not knowing the cause of their symptoms, may become very concerned, are often shunted from one hospital department to another, go through endless investigations, eluding specialist after specialist, until an astute physician spots the breathing pattern. Sometimes hyperventilation alternates with hypoventilation because a nervous stimulus for breathing is the acidic reaction of the blood. When hyperventilation causes blood to be alkaline, the brain center responsible for breathing becomes inactive, nature's way of restoring the acidity of the blood. If this pattern is constantly repeated, as it often is in chronic anxious hyperventilators, the body is rarely functioning in an ideal way and chronic tiredness or one of numerous psychosomatic disorders is the result. It is important that we understand the relationship between emotion, breathing, and the autonomic nervous system if we are to prevent illness and promote positive health.

Sleep Apnea

Sleep apnea has recently received much attention. In this type of breathing, there is a sudden and temporary cessation of breathing at any point in the inhalation-exhalation cycle. Such interruptions can occur during day or night although it is night apnea that has received most attention. Typically, periodically throughout the night, the individual stops breathing, from a few seconds to a minute. This apnea seems to have serious implications for health, for breathing pauses are often accompanied by a rise in blood pressure and a decrease in the level of blood oxygen, which may fall to such a low level that the individual may in fact turn blue for a few seconds. In one study, the blood pressure of half the subjects rose and remained raised throughout the day (107). These people also have a tendency to anxiety, depression, and confusion; a decreased sexual drive; and an increased propensity to develop coronary heart disease.

In another study a number of ordinary hospital patients were examined and two-thirds of the men were found to have periods of apnea associated with lowering of blood oxygen levels lasting longer than ten seconds. Oddly enough, a very small number of women experienced sleep apnea and none of these were associated with low levels of blood oxygen (46). The deleterious effect of sleep apnea is compound. A rise in blood pressure means that the work of the heart is increased since it has to pump blood against the higher pressure. On the other hand, the blood level of oxygen is decreased, thus creating a further relative deficiency of oxygen.

If this temporary energy shortage is repeated several times a night for a number of years, the cumulative effect on the heart's functioning could be considerable. Since the death rate from heart disease is two to three times higher in men than in women we might ask: Could this difference in rate be related to sleep apnea in any way? Could a modification of breathing patterns prevent heart disease? We do not know the answer at present.

Paradoxical Breathing

In this type of breathing, both diaphragm and abdominal muscles are contracted at the same time. It is as if the individual is preparing to receive a blow. In a real situation the contraction of abdominal muscles will render the wall rigid, so that it protects the internal organs. But a danger that is in a person's mind tends to counteract breathing efforts. During inhalation the diaphragm moves downward to let the lungs expand and accommodate inhaled breath. If the abdominal muscles contract at the same time they will push the internal organs and the diaphragm upward at the same time, thus making inhalation weak and inefficient.

BREATHING EXERCISE

It is worth taking some time off to master proper diaphragmatic exercise. Follow Practice 1 first. If you are not quite sure that you are doing the exercise correctly or if you are having difficulty with this method, try the second method, in which you lie on your stomach. Only when you have mastered diaphragmatic breathing should you go on to try alternate-nostril breathing. Once you have learned the technique you should be able to restore the pattern in one breath and relax your body at the same time, which is the ultimate long-term goal.

Practice 1: Abdominal Breathing Exercise: Supine Position

1. Lie on your back with your feet a comfortable distance apart or sit upright comfortably, but not rigidly.
2. Close your eyes.
3. Place one hand on your chest and the other on your abdomen. Become aware of the rate and rhythm of your breath. Note which hand is moving with your breathing movements.

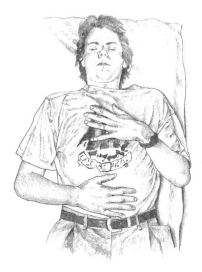

4. Inhale and exhale slowly, smoothly, and deeply through the nostrils without noise, jerks, or pauses.
5. Consciously pull your abdominal muscles in when you exhale and, if necessary, push the abdominal muscles gently with your hand. When you breathe in be aware of the abdominal wall pushing out.
6. Now place your hands by your side, continue inhaling and exhaling, and concentrate exclusively on the breathing movements, being aware only of your abdomen rising and falling.
7. Just become aware of the rhythm of inhalation and exhalation. Normally we breath about twelve to sixteen times a minute when we are resting. As your mind becomes calmer you will notice that your breathing becomes slower.
8. Practice for three to five minutes a day until you clearly understand the movement, and diaphragmatic breathing becomes your natural pattern of breathing, whether you are sitting, standing or lying down.

Practice 2: Abdominal Breathing Exercise: Crocodile Position

1. Lie on your stomach, and place your legs a comfortable distance apart with your toes pointing outwards.

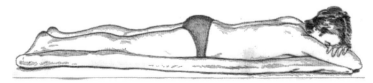

2. Fold your arms in front of your body, resting your hands on your biceps. Position your arms so that your chest does not touch the floor. This position necessitates diaphragmatic breathing.
3. Inhale and exhale slowly, smoothly, and deeply through the nostrils without noise, jerks or pauses.
4. When you inhale, feel your abdomen pressing against the floor, and when you exhale, feel your abdominal muscles lifting off the floor.
5. Just become aware of this rhythmical movement of the diaphragm and alternate pressing of the abdomen against the floor.
6. Practice for three to five minutes a day until you feel that diaphragmatic breathing is easy whether you are sitting or standing.

Practice 3: Alternate-Nostril Breathing

1. Sit in a comfortable position with your head, neck, and trunk relatively erect.
2. Breathe slowly and gently using the diaphragm as described in the earlier practices. There should be no sound, jerks, or pauses.

3. With your right thumb pressing gently on the right nostril, slowly exhale and then slowly inhale through the left nostril.

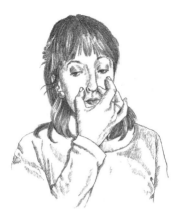

4. Now lift your thumb to open the right nostril and with your middle finger gently press the left nostril. Slowly exhale and then slowly inhale through the right nostril.
5. Repeat the cycle six times so that a complete cycle of exhalation and inhalation through each nostril is carried out three times. This cycle of six breaths completes one "round."
6. Now breathe through both nostrils three times.
7. Repeat two more rounds interposing normal breathing through both nostrils between each round. There will be a total of nine complete breaths through each nostril.
8. A good time to practice this is every evening before going to sleep. If possible, repeat in the morning as well.

Practice 4: Revitalizing Breath

Oxygen taken during each inspiration revitalizes every single cell in the body.

Try to imagine this process actually taking place. Through this imagination you can send energy-giving breath to any area which feels dull or sluggish.

1. You can do this exercise sitting down or standing up. Close your eyes if you like.
2. Take a deep breath in and feel your abdomen expand as you bring your arms out in front of you and slowly up over your head.
3. Stretch as you breathe out and slowly bring down your arms.
4. As you breathe in again, imagine your breath revitalizing your entire body, filling it with energy and dissolving away the tension. Feel it becoming alive with oxygen spreading through every part of your body as you bring your arms up again as in Number 2 above.
5. Slowly exhale and bring your arms down by your side.
6. Repeat the above sequence three times. Notice any sensations you may feel, for example, warmth, relaxation, or tingling.
7. Now focus on an area where you feel tension, for example, between your shoulder blades. Take another, revitalizing, deep breath and feel it moving into the tense area. Imagine your warm breath massaging the area and easing away the tension. Exhale.
8. Choose another tense area to focus on and repeat the exercise.
9. Take a few inspirations and expirations and imagine your body full of vigor and vitality.
10. Stretch slowly as your palms reach up toward the ceiling and rock your body from side to side by switching your weight from your left foot to your right foot. Slowly bring your arms down to your sides.

11. Stand still for a few seconds and enjoy the sights and colors around you. Continue with your routine, feeling refreshed and happy.
12. Practice twice a day for about three minutes each time.

ONE-BREATH MINIRELAXATION

Several times during the day become aware of your breathing. Just take one deep breath and feel the energy coming in and revitalizing your body. Breathe out and relax. Use frequent occurrences in your daily life like a telephone ringing, getting in or out of the car, stopping at red traffic lights while driving, waiting before meetings, or between different tasks. You should be able to fit in approximately twenty such one-breath relaxation exercises during your entire day. This exercise is discussed more fully in the next chapter under the heading "Integrating Relaxation into Everyday Life."

10

Physical Relaxation

We all need to develop some sort of mechanism for relaxing and coping with stress. Simple forms of relaxation which many people intuitively use are listed below. Tick those which you regularly use. Add those which do not appear on the list.

EXAMPLES OF SIMPLE RELAXATION

- Listen to music.
- Go for a walk.
- Play a game of tennis, golf, or other sport.
- Go for a leisurely swim.
- Engage in an active, absorbing hobby.
- Play solitaire.
- Have a hot bath.
- Visit a friend.
- Play with children.
- Go to the theater or the movies.
- Watch television.
- Sip a long drink.
- Lie in the sun.

- Read a good book.
- Do keep-fit exercises.
- Practice Yoga.
- Have a snooze.
- Do gardening.
- Look at family photo albums or holiday snaps.
- Have your hair done.
- Enjoy a sauna or Turkish bath.
- Go mushroom or berry picking.
- Visit an art gallery.
- Buy a record.
- Go dancing.
- Have dinner in a restaurant.
- Just sit and do nothing.
- Go on a picnic.
- Do a crossword puzzle.

RELAXATION TRAINING

It is difficult to feel or act at ease when the body is tense. Medical research shows that chronic muscle tension contributes to a variety of health problems. Releasing both mental and physical tension can bring many benefits, including lowering of blood pressure, reducing the risk of coronary heart disease, improving the quality of sleep, and bringing a certain degree of relief from migraine, tension headaches, arthritic pain, anxiety, sexual dysfunction, and other psychosomatic disorders. Certainly no method is a cure-all and not everyone gets the same amount of benefit. However, most people who regularly practice relaxation experience general improvement in their sense of sell-being. Unfortunately, most of our tension remains undetected because the brain pushes the information coming from the body into the subconscious if it is constantly bombarded with that information, particularly if it is also kept busy with pursuing daily jobs which have been given top priority.

Relaxation, both mental and physical, means much more than simply sitting down and "taking it easy." It is a skill, like driving a car, and it has to be learned until, again like driving a car, it becomes second nature. Like the learning of any new skill, relaxation training requires three things: motivation, understanding, and commitment. You must be motivated to learn; unless and until you genuinely want to learn yourself, no amount of advice will be sufficient for you to develop the skill. Once motivated, you must gain an understanding of what you are trying to achieve, what are the principles involved, and why relaxation is likely to help you. Finally, there must be a commitment to continue using the skill on a regular basis. There must be a strong desire to take control of your health. Learning relaxation is not very difficult. The most difficult aspect is to discipline yourself to comply with it over the long run.

DEEP MUSCLE RELAXATION

Each time one of your muscles contracts, thousands of electrical impulses travel along the nerves to the brain. There is scientific evidence which suggests that a part of the brain called the *hypothalamus*, which controls the stress response with its mental, emotional, behavioral, and physical components, becomes highly charged when it is bombarded with a variety of sensory stimulations. When the hypothalamus is sensitized in this way, everyday stressors can easily lead to a stress response. It is possible to cut down drastically on the sensory impulses traveling to the brain simply by lying down, closing your eyes, learning not to be distracted by external noises, and then deeply relaxing the entire body. The result is amazing: both body and mind return to a state of balance or recuperative rest.

Such relaxation should occur spontaneously after any activity but, unfortunately, the endless demands of modern life often prevent this. The result is an accumulated state of stress which can eventually culminate in a stress disorder. You need to learn the art of letting go and allowing your body's restorative ability to take over. If relaxation is to be effective there are a number of general conditions you must consider before getting down to practice.

Time

Deep muscle relaxation is most beneficial if it is carried out twice a day with at least three to four hours and preferably eight to ten hours between. This would most suitably be in the morning and evening. If it is impossible to have two periods, one may do, in which case choose the time immediately after work before spending your time with the family. A recuperative period after work means plenty of energy and maximum enjoyment in the evening. Avoid leaving the practice until late in the evening, as many people tend to fall asleep and then wake up in the middle of the night. It is not a good idea to practice immediately after a meal as sudden relaxation of the stomach may occur, which may interfere with digestion and may occasionally give you nausea. As a general rule, allow half an hour after a snack, one hour after a light meal, and two hours after a heavy meal.

Place

It is essential to have a quiet, warm, comfortable place which affords privacy. There should be no bright lights glaring at you. The fewer the distractions, the better your practice will be. If the phone is likely to ring it may be a good idea to take it off the hook. The radio and television should be turned of, and make an agreement with your family that they should not disturb you for half an hour. Alternatively, let your family join you in the practice. If finding a quiet place at home is impossible, you might consider staying at work after hours. If that, too, is difficult, go to the public library reading room, which will be quiet, but you will have to make do with sitting in whatever type of chair is available.

Posture

Deep muscle relaxation can be practiced lying on a firm bed or on the floor. Alternatively, it can be practiced sitting in a comfortable armchair with a high back which can support your own back, neck, and head. It should be large enough to support your buttocks and thighs. Make sure you are comfortable, in loose-fitting garments. Loosen your tie, belt, and other constricting clothes.

If lying flat on your back, make sure that your head, neck, and trunk are in a straight line. Keep your legs a little apart so that your feet are approximately one and a half feet apart, allow your feet to flop loosely, with your toes pointing outward and your heels pointing inward. If you are not used to lying flat you may find this position somewhat uncomfortable. If so, use a small pillow under your head and a folded towel or cushion behind your knees or under your back. The important thing is to be sure that you are comfortable; otherwise you will find it difficult to relax deeply.

Instructions for Deep Muscle Relaxation

Follow the relaxation instructions given below. Read the instructions several times before starting the practice. Better still is having a friend or spouse read the instructions slowly in a monotonous voice while you follow them. Alternatively, record the instructions on a cassette and then practice while you listen to it. As any relaxation must start with a diaphragmatic breathing exercise, the instructions will begin with a breathing exercise. The method is based on yogic exercise. I have used these instructions for the last twenty years in a variety of conditions and have found them most acceptable to the patients. In a number of scientific studies my colleagues and I have carried out (99-104), they have shown efficacy in reducing high blood pressure and risk of having a heart attack in the future in addition to increasing a sense of well-being and an improved quality of life. The instructions start with yogic maximum breath followed by diaphragmatic breathing and then deep muscle relaxation. Our complete program also includes mental relaxation and various intellectual strategies, which will be found in subsequent chapters.

- Make sure your head, body, and legs are in a straight line. Keep your legs a little apart and allow your feet to flop loosely so that your heels are pointing inward and your toes are pointing outward. Keep your hands by your sides with the palms upward and the fingers slightly flexed.

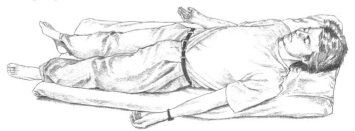

- Close your eyes. Very slowly fill your lungs, starting at the diaphragm and working right up to the top of the chest; then very slowly breathe out. After three slow maximum breaths, allow your breathing to become normal and regular. Breathe in and out gently and rhythmically, using your diaphragm. Don't force your breath. Don't try to make it slow deliberately. Just keep your own rhythm. Be completely aware of your breathing pattern. Feel the subtle difference in the temperature of the air you are inhaling and the air you are exhaling. The air you breathe in is cooler and the air you breathe out is warmer.

- Now you are consciously going to relax each part of the body in turn. Relaxation means the complete absence of movement, since even the slightest movement means that some of your muscles are contracting. It is also not holding any part rigid. Concentrate on the part you are relaxing.

- Now take your mind to your right foot and relax your toes, instep, heel, and ankle; stay there for a few seconds. Now move your attention slowly up, relaxing your leg, calf, knee, thigh, and hip. Feel all the muscles, joints, and tissues of your right leg becoming completely relaxed. Relax as deeply as you can. Just keep your awareness on this feeling of deep relaxation in your right leg for a few moments.

- Now take your mind to your left foot and repeat the process, working up the leg, thigh, and hip as before. Let all the tension ease away and enjoy the feeling of relaxation for a few seconds.

- Next concentrate on your right hand. Relax the fingers, thumb, palm, and wrist. Move your attention up to your forearm, elbow, upper arm, and shoulder. Feel every muscle, joint, and tissue in your right arm becoming deeply relaxed. Fix your attention on the sensation of relaxation in your entire right arm for a few moments.

- Now become aware of your left hand and relax the fingers, thumb, palm, wrist, forearm, elbow, upper arm, and shoulder. Let all the tension ease away from the left arm.

- Now concentrate on the base of your spine, vertebra by vertebra, relaxing each vertebra and the muscles on either side of the spine into the floor. Relax your back, first the lower back, then the middle back, and finally the upper back. Release all the tension from your back. Let the relaxation become deeper and deeper, feel the back merging with the floor.

- Let the muscles in your neck relax next. Let all the muscles in the front of your neck relax. Let your head rest gently and feel the back of the neck relaxing. Let the relaxation become as deep as possible.

- Relax your chest. Every time you breathe out relax a little more. Let your body sink into the floor a little more each time. Let all the nerves, muscles, and organs in your chest relax completely. Now relax the muscles of your stomach. Let all the nerves, muscles, and organs in your stomach relax completely. Just think as if they are relaxing.

- Now concentrate on your jaw. Let it relax so that it drops slightly. Your lips are just touching each other and your teeth are apart. Relax your tongue; relax the muscles around your cheek bones. Relax your eyes and the muscles around your eyes. Feel them becoming relaxed. Your eyes must become very, very still. Now relax your forehead; let all the muscles in your forehead become completely relaxed. There is no tension in your facial muscles at all. Now relax your scalp and all the muscles around your head. Your body is now completely relaxed. Keep it relaxed for five more minutes.

Coming Out of Relaxation

To come out of relaxation, take one deep breath, and feel the energy coming down into your arms and legs. Move your arms and legs slowly. Open your eyes without reacting to the light, and slowly sit up. Stretch your body, and feel refreshed and reenergized.

Integrating Relaxation into Everyday Life

Once you have mastered the technique you should be able to relax when appropriate—sitting, standing, or lying down—and within a matter of seconds. Breathing exercise and relaxation techniques are not just rituals to be practiced once or twice a day. They are meant to change our attitudes and the way we cope with our everyday stress. Most of our stress does not come in big packages. Of course, bereavement, getting married, or being fired after twenty years of service are likely to cause major distress, but we often forget that it is the little insults of everyday life—the irritation caused by the so-called trivia, like traffic jams, being interrupted by numerous telephone calls when we are trying to finish some important paperwork, being under constant time pressure, not being appreciated for our good work, having the roof start leaking as we get ready to go to work, waiting for a babysitter who doesn't show up, having someone spill beer on our sofa, and having to put up with an incompetent shop assistant—that accumulate and take a major toll on our health and well-being.

I recommend that you practice brief relaxations several times a day so that stress does not accumulate to the point where it causes distress or stress symptoms. For example, every time you come across a red traffic light when driving a car, release your grip on the steering wheel, take one deep breath, and let body relax. It does not matter whether it is five seconds or twenty-five seconds. A little relaxation practiced often ensures that tension will not build up to the degree that makes us feel like swearing. Driving often brings out the animal instinct in us, and car manufacturers often take advantage of this fact and try to appeal to our primitive instincts by naming cars Jaguar, Mustang, Hawk, Rapier, Scepter, Avenger, Hunter, and so on, and one oil company urges us to put nothing less than a tiger in our tank!

Another helpful suggestion is to practice a similar brief relaxation before you pick up a phone that is ringing. You will find that by doing this not only will you practice mini-relaxation several times a day, but also your interaction with the person at the other end of the telephone line will be much more calm and friendly. Another good idea is to stick a little colored dot on your wristwatch dial so that every time you look at the watch, which is usually when you are under time pressure, you are reminded to practice your one-breath relaxation. If you are late there is nothing you can do about it, and if you compose yourself by doing a brief relaxation, rather than expending your energy in worrying about it, it is quite possible that you will be more likely to achieve your goal.

Make a list of ten situations in your life that are likely to make you tense or upset and then try to relax briefly before or during them, trying with minor situations first and then going on to more difficult ones. It will be commendable if you can manage to integrate about twenty such brief relaxations into your ordinary day.

PROGRESSIVE MUSCLE RELAXATION

The technique of progressive muscle relaxation was developed by an American physician, Edmund Jacobson (60). It is similar to deep muscle relaxation, except that you first tense each group of muscles before relaxing them. The logic behind tensing the muscle before relaxing it is that this helps to focus attention on the feeling of tension in the body. The more aware you are of tension, the easier it is to control. The degree of tightening required varies according to how tense you already are. Someone who is very tense to start with will have to tighten extremely hard to notice the tension. As a general rule you are asked to squeeze firmly and maintain that tension for five to seven seconds. Tensing too hard or too long can give you cramps or pain and should be avoided. Tension in muscles also raises your blood pressure considerably. For those who already have high blood pressure I personally do not advise progressive muscle relaxation as I believe that the best results can be achieved by combining diaphragmatic breathing exercise with deep muscle relaxation and, if possible, a simple form of meditation. For other problems (anxiety states, for example), progressive muscle relaxation is quite suitable.

When you let go of tension, do it quickly so that the muscles relax immediately and you are able to distinguish between the feelings of relaxation and of tension quite easily. It is important not to hold your breath while doing the exercise. You may find this somewhat difficult to start with as tensing of any group of muscles automatically makes you tense your chest muscles. However, with practice it becomes easier to tense all the group of muscles that you are asked to tense while keeping the rest of the body in a relaxed position and breathing regularly. It is also helpful to coordinate your breath in such a way that you breathe in just before you tense the muscles and you breathe out when you let go of tension. No special way of breathing is recommended except that you breathe in a very passive way without making any conscious efforts to regulate your breathing in any way. It is likely that as your body relaxes the breathing pattern will automatically become deep and regular.

As with all forms of relaxation, it is important that you pay careful attention to whatever you are doing in the exercise, relaxing or tensing. Like deep muscle relaxation, progressive muscle relaxation should be practiced twice a day. It should be practiced before a meal or after a suitable interval following a meal according to the general rules suggested under deep muscle relaxation. It is best practiced while sitting in a comfortable armchair with a high back. Dr. Jacobson took several months to train an individual in progressive muscle relaxation. The following is a shortened, more modern version of the technique.

Session One

1. Tense your right arm; make a fist and then tighten your upper arm.

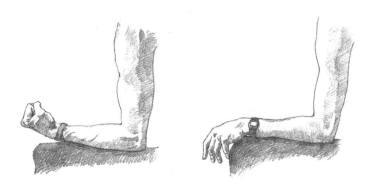

2. Hold the tension for five to seven seconds.
3. Release the tension as you exhale. Relax for twenty to thirty seconds.
4. Repeat 1-3 above.
5. Tense your left arm; make a fist and then tighten your entire left arm.
6. Hold the tension for five to seven seconds.
7. Release the tension as you exhale. Relax for twenty to thirty seconds.
8. Repeat 5-7 above.
9. Tense your chest, back, and shoulders. Take a deep breath, hold it, and try to bring your shoulder blades together by pressing hard. Tighten your chest muscles at the same time.
10. Hold the tense position for five to seven seconds.
11. Release the tension and breathe out. Relax for twenty to thirty seconds.
12. Repeat 9-11 above.

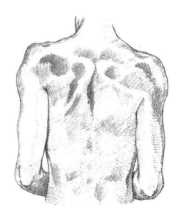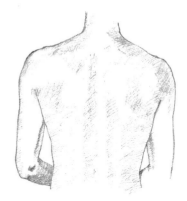

Session Two

After one week of practicing Session One, proceed to the second session. The following is a suggested sequence for all thirteen groups of muscles. Practice as many as you can manage comfortably. Make sure that you are mastering the technique properly before going on to the next group of muscles.

1. Right arm, tense and relax
2. Left arm, tense and relax
3. Right leg, tense and relax

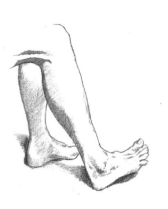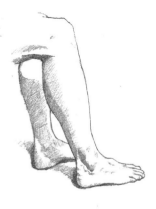

4. Left leg, tense and relax
5. Pelvis, tighten and relax
6. Abdomen, tense and relax
7. Breathe into chest; hold the breath and then relax
8. Back and shoulders, tighten and relax
9. Clench jaws and relax
10. Purse lips and relax
11. Eye muscles, tense (screw up tight) and relax

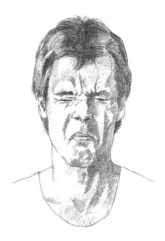

12. Forehead, tense (frown) and relax
13. Tense entire body and relax

Session Three

In this session, instead of tensing and relaxing individual groups of muscles separately, you combine them into four groups as follows.

1. Right arm and left arm
2. Head and neck including forehead, nose, cheeks, jaw, and tongue

3. Shoulders, back, and chest as well as abdomen
4. Right leg and left leg

Session Four

In this session, instead of relaxing and tensing each group of muscles, you just relax them. Continue practicing once or twice a day.

AUTOGENIC TRAINING

The fact that we can bring about relaxation in our bodies by thinking in a certain way was noted by several physicians at the beginning of the twentieth century. Autogenic means self-generating. *Autogenic* training was developed by a German psychiatrist, Johannes Schultz, and was popularized in the West by Wolfgang Luthe (75). It consists of a series of phrases which people repeat to themselves mentally, giving self- or autosuggestion. These phrases are based on three physiological states: a sensation of heaviness in the limbs, a feeling of warmth, and easy, natural breathing. The suggestion of heaviness in the limbs actually leads to the feeling of heaviness associated with relaxation. About 10 percent of people fail to feel heaviness although their limbs do relax. The suggestion of warmth is quite logical since one of the effects of the stress response is cooling of the skin because of the constriction of blood vessels which is necessary to help divert blood to where it is needed most, the brain and the muscles. As discussed earlier, breathing becomes erratic during the stress response. It may become quicker and deeper, or if the chest muscles are tense, it may become shallow, and in extreme cases hyperventilation may occur. By suggesting repeatedly that breathing is relaxed, it may actually become natural and rhythmical.

Autogenic exercise can be self-taught, but it is better to learn under the supervision of a qualified teacher as it can sometimes cause adverse reactions, such as acute anxiety, palpitations, or rapid breathing. Asthma or peptic ulcer symptoms can be made worse by the solar plexus formula (see below).

Time

It is recommended that you practice this exercise three to four times a day. The best times are early in the morning, before breakfast, during your coffee break, before lunch, before supper, or in bed before going to sleep.

Place

It should be practiced in a place that is quiet, warm, and comfortable. You may want to take the phone off the hook and turn off the radio or television. If it is difficult to find a place where you can be alone, it can be carried out in a bathroom or even on the toilet!

Attitude

Your attitude should be passive. If your mind wanders away from the exercise to other thoughts, don't be impatient or irritable. Just let your attention return to the exercise as soon as you realize that your mind has drifted elsewhere. Don't get involved with the actual meaning of phrases or feel upset that you are feeling light instead of heavy or feeling cold instead of warm.

Posture

You can lie on your back as described in the previous relaxation exercises or sit in an armchair with a high back that can support your head. Even if you are sitting on a stool, it is quite all right to practice autogenic training provided that your weight is distributed evenly and both right and left sides are balanced. Your legs must be uncrossed, your feet should be placed flat on the ground, and your arms should be partially bent and supported on your thighs or in your lap.

Session One

Close your eyes and repeat to yourself mentally the following phrases. This session should be restricted to heaviness phrases as follows:

- My right arm is heavy.
- My left arm is heavy.
- Both my arms are heavy.
- My right leg is heavy.
- My left leg is heavy.
- Both my legs are heavy.
- My arms and legs are heavy.

You can either use one phrase to start with or repeat all of them, depending on how comfortable you feel. If you use only one phrase, the whole exercise will last twenty to thirty seconds, but if you use all the phrases above, it may take between three and five minutes. Repeat each phrase three times and allow a few seconds before going on to the next phrase, and imagine the feelings which are suggested.

Session Two

This session should be undertaken after you have been practicing Session One for a few days and you or your therapist feels satisfied with the progress you have made. In this session we use the phrases based on the feeling of warmth, as

- My right arm is warm.

- My left arm is warm.
- Both my arms are warm.
- My right leg is warm.
- My left leg is warm.
- Both my legs are warm.
- My arms and legs are warm.

You practice heaviness phrases first followed by the above warmth phrases. Again use as many as you feel comfortable with at first and progress until you can use all the warmth phrases before going on to Session Three. If you repeat each of the Session One and Session Two phrases three times with pauses in between, it should take between seven and ten minutes to complete the exercise. Practice the entire exercise three times a day. If you feel unduly warm during the exercise, insert the word *comfortably* before *warm*. For example, "My right arm is comfortably warm." You can also add a new phrase, "My neck and shoulders are heavy," and use this new phrase during daily life as well, for example, when you are waiting at a red traffic light while driving.

Possible Unexpected Sensations

Many people experience novel sensations such as the following:

- Feeling of detachment in one limb.
- Feeling of numbness or tingling in one or more limbs.
- Twitching sensation anywhere in the body.
- Feeling of weakness.
- Floating sensation.
- Feeling that one arm is bigger than the other.

Don't let these sensations worry you. They are perfectly normal and quite intriguing once you become familiar with them.

Session Three

This session is concerned with breathing. The phrase for this exercise is "My body breathes me." Repeat all the phrases of Sessions One and Two three times followed by the breathing phrase above. Repeat it several times before ending the session by repeating, "My neck and shoulders are heavy." Practice the entire exercise twice a day and practice minirelaxation several times a day when you just repeat, "My neck and shoulders are heavy," three to five times or more. Continue practicing in this manner for a week or two before going on to Session Four.

Session Four

This session uses a new phrase, "My forehead is cool and relaxed." When people get upset, they often feel flushed in the face. The new phrase can bring the soothing feeling of a cool, damp flannel across the forehead. As in other sessions, you should repeat all the phrases of previous sessions before going on to this phrase; actually try to feel what is suggested. Continue practicing the entire session once or twice a day, with minisessions three to five times a day. If you do not have sufficient time you can shorten the exercise by combining phrases and repeating them only once or twice, for example:

- My right arm is heavy—repeat once.
- My arms and legs are heavy—repeat three times.
- My arms and legs are warm—repeat three times.
- My body breathes me—repeat three times.
- My neck and shoulders are heavy—repeat once.

Continue practicing these regularly. The phrases for the fifth and sixth sessions are "My heartbeat is calm and regular" and "My solar plexus (center of the abdomen) is warm," but they are better left alone if you do not have a therapist to supervise you.

Autogenic training can be taken further than the basic six formulae to include meditation or mental formulae such as:

- My mind is calm and serene.
- I am at peace.

MASSAGE

In the formal sense, massage includes deliberate, purposeful manipulation of either part or the whole of the body. Informally, it also includes vigorous rubbing, gentle stroking, or even kissing to ease pain or anxiety. We often say to a child who is hurt, "Let me rub it better or kiss it better." Being massaged is enjoyable and relaxing. The human touch brings feelings of warmth and of being cared for. These greatly increase our sense of well-being. Massage also stimulates the circulation, which both brings a fresh supply of fuel to all parts of the body and removes accumulated toxic wastes. It helps fluid drainage and can reduce swelling. Stiff muscles or joints can be made more mobile with appropriate massage. It is often an effective treatment in sports medicine.

The art of giving massage lies in knowing which part of the hand to use and how much pressure to apply for each movement, and this can be learned only through practice. It is important that your hands be kept in constant contact with your partner's body and that you maintain a regular rhythm. Stopping and starting, or lifting your hands in the middle, interrupt the rhythm and destroy the effect. Giving someone a massage using some of the best-known massage techniques (stroking, pummeling, kneading, circular pressure, and percussion movement) can be relaxing for both the giver and the recipient of the massage. You can benefit either by reading a detailed book (85) on massage or, better still, by attending a short course.

Basic Movements

Stroking. The hands are placed on the part to be massaged and then moved in a sweeping circular fashion, slowly and rhythmically, with more pressure being applied when stroking toward the heart. The pressure may be light or deep and the rate may be quick or slow, but it is important not to lose touch or the rhythm. Stroking is usually used for large areas like the back, thigh, or calf.

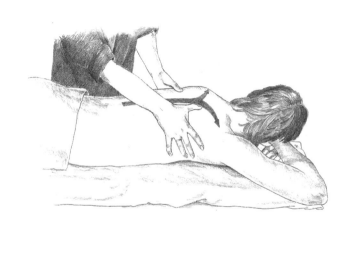

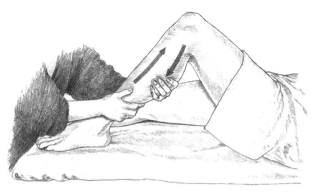

Kneading or Petrissage. This involves firm manipulation by the hands in a semicircular fashion, either in the same or in opposite directions. If the area to be massaged is small, the same movements can be performed by the fingertips or the thumbs. The buttocks, thighs, and shoulders are suitable areas for this movement. In self-massage one or both hands can be used for rolling, squeezing, or pressing movements.

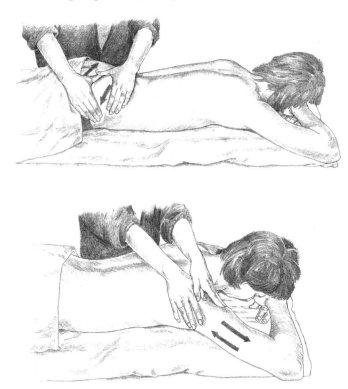

Pressure. This is a form of finger kneading, popular in a Japanese technique known as *shiatsu*. It uses gentle pressure with the thumbs to improve circulation. It can be used, for example, on either side of the spine.

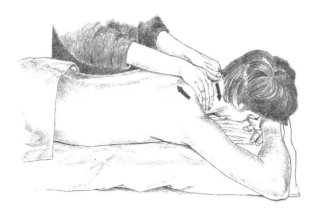

Friction. This involves a localized rubbing action for areas which feel tense, knotty, or stringy such as the shoulders, the back of the neck, or the temples. Press down with the pads of one or more fingers, the thumb, or the heel of your hand and give a deep circular massage for about three to four seconds and then repeat the movement.

Self-Massage

It is very difficult to relax while massaging yourself as some of your muscles will be working and, therefore, inevitably tense. You can, however, massage any specific area that feels tense, such as your scalp, the back of your neck, your temples, shoulders, hands, lower back, calves, and feet. Self-massage is particularly helpful in relieving aches and pains accumulated during the day, such as a headache or tired feet. It is better if you can work directly on the skin but it is not necessary to remove your clothes except perhaps your jacket and your shoes if you are working on your feet. Massaging while having a bath or watching television is ideal. Use a little pleasant-smelling oil to lubricate your skin if you can.

The following are suggested movements for specific areas.

Face. Sit yourself comfortably and hold your palms over your eyes. This helps you to focus on yourself. After a few seconds, move your hands up to your forehead and stroke firmly with your fingertips from the center outward several times.

Place one or two fingertips on your temples and gently rub or use circular pressing movements. After a few seconds on each spot move your fingertips up or down or behind a little and repeat the movements.

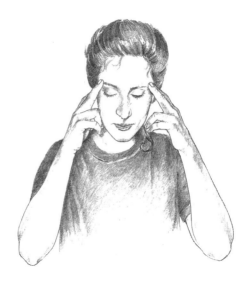

Scalp and Neck. Spread out your fingertips over your scalp, press firmly, and try to move your scalp up and down on your skull.

Now place the middle three fingers of each hand on either side of your spine, starting just below your head, and firmly stroke outward for a few seconds. Move your fingertips lower down and repeat the movements until you have covered your entire neck.

Shoulders. Place your hands over the top of the opposite shoulder and, using firm squeezing movements, knead the muscles from the side of the neck to the upper arms. You can also grasp the bulky muscle in your hand and then move your

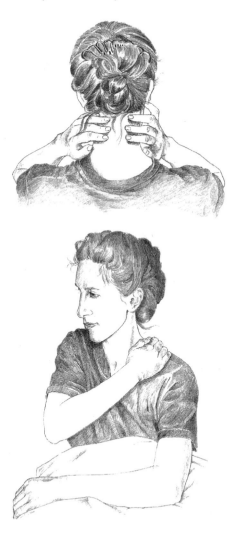

upper arm in a circular fashion. If there is a lot of tension, use localized rubbing with several fingertips.

Back. Place your hands on either side of your lower back with your fingers or fists pointing downward and make deep stroking movements outward several times. Repeat the movement after moving your hands gradually upward. Use kneading movements and squeeze the small of your back on either side.

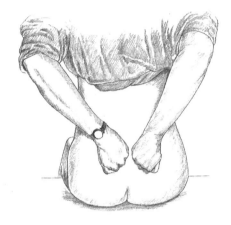

Hands and Arms. Hold your right hand palm upward in your left-hand fingers and palm and, with your left-hand thumb, rub or apply circular pressing movements to various areas of the right palm and the wrist. Using squeezing movements, knead your fingers and thumb up and down. Now turn your hand palm downward and rub your knuckles and all the areas on the back of your right hand and wrist. You may also stroke across the back of your hand and wrist with the heel of your hand and repeat the movement as you move a little further up each time, thus covering the entire arm. Kneading can also be used for the upper arms. Repeat on the other side.

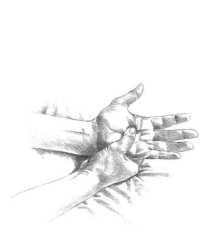

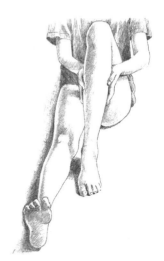

Legs and Thighs. Sit on the floor. Bend your right knee with your foot resting firmly on the ground. Start low down on the calf and work gradually upward as far as you can go on the back of your thigh. Stroke deeply upward and outward with both hands. Rub with your thumbs or fingertips to relieve localized tension. Grasp your Achilles' tendon between your thumb and fingers. Rub by moving your fingers and your thumb in the opposite directions. Repeat on the other side.

Feet. Rest your right ankle over your left knee. Hold your foot in one hand and with the thumb of the other hand rub the entire sole, moving your thumb little by little after three to four seconds of rubbing over each spot. In addition, give deep strokes with the heel of your right hand while support-

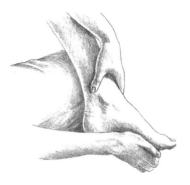

ing the foot in your left hand. Grasp each toe between a thumb
and an index finger. Pull it toward you and stretch the muscles
and tendons. Repeat on the other foot.

BIOFEEDBACK

Biofeedback treatment is a way of regulating deranged biological functions by connecting you to electronic instruments,
usually by means of electrode wires attached to appropriate
parts of the body, which then measure a variety of physiological
functions and display them by means of visual or sound signals.
Skin temperature, sweat gland activity, the level of tension in
the muscles, blood pressure, heart rate, and the electrical activity of the brain are examples of the functions which can be
measured and displayed in these ways. You then try to change
the function, by subjective mental processes, in the desired direction. Any change in the physical function is immediately obvious by an appropriate change in the visual or sound signals.
The idea behind this procedure is that knowledge of success
reinforces the learning. As the person begins to make progress,
his task is made more and more difficult until satisfactory progress is made and the person feels confident in regulating the
function in question, without the help of the instruments. Mental and physical relaxation techniques are often used by the
subject to restore normality.

I often use an instrument measuring galvanic skin resistance
(GSR), which basically measures sweat gland activity, in my
behavioral program to reduce high blood pressure. People often
break out in sweats when frightened or angry. Such emotional
states also tend to raise blood pressure. When we become relaxed, sweat gland activity becomes lower and the sound signal
becomes fainter and fainter and eventually stops. When that
happens, the frequency of the machine is turned up and another sound signal is delivered, and the patient has to relax

deeper before the signal can be turned off. His task of switching off the signal gets harder as he gets better in the relaxation skill. Even though there is no direct or proportional relationship between sweat gland activity and blood pressure, by learning to control sweat gland activity we can indirectly learn to control blood pressure. The reasons for using this instrument, rather than a blood pressure biofeedback, are its simplicity and cheapness. Training in abdominal breathing exercises, in the deep muscle relaxation already described, and in visualization and meditation helps people to learn biofeedback control of both sweat gland activity and blood pressure.

Similar programs are available for sufferers of tension headaches, migraine, insomnia, and other stress-related symptoms or disorders, although the types of instruments used vary somewhat. For example, thermal or temperature control feedback is often used for migraine sufferers. This practice originated from the observation that many migraine patients notice coldness of their fingers before the headache starts. By learning to raise the temperature of the hands, the patient frequently is able to avert an attack of headache. On the other hand, electromyograph (EMG) biofeedback is often used in the treatment of tension headaches. EMG measures the level of tension in the muscles over which the electrodes are applied, and the task to learn is to lower the tension by relaxing those muscles.

11

Mental Relaxation

MEDITATION

Meditation has been a part of most cultures and religions, both Eastern and Western, throughout the ages. The meditation methods described in various branches of Yoga are probably the oldest, while Christian prayer, Jewish meditation, Japanese Zen, Chinese Tao, Muslim Sufism, and the meditation of Hinduism and Buddhism are some other examples. Only recently, however, have medical people realized that it can be used, without any religious connotation, in the promotion of health. As a result, several hundred papers and books have appeared in the medical literature, describing the physiological and psychological effects of meditation as well as the physical, emotional, and spiritual well-being of its practitioners.

First, meditation practice involves taking a comfortable position; either sitting, lying down, or standing, although sitting is the most usual posture. Second, it must take place in a quiet environment. Third, the practitioner regulates his breath, adopting a physically relaxed and mentally passive attitude, and finally he dwells single-mindedly upon an object (8, 53, 70). The object of meditation does not have to be physical. It can be an idea, image, or happening; it can be mental repetition of a word or phrase as in mantra meditation; it can be observing our own thoughts, perceptions, or reactions; or it can be concentrating on some bodily generated rhythms like breathing. In religious practice, needless to say, the object of concentration is God.

The multiplicity of the objects upon which we can meditate allows for individual variations. People differ in their intellectual and emotional makeup, and it is important that the person feels comfortable with the object chosen. The ultimate idea is to learn the discipline of concentrating on one thing and only one thing at a time, to the exclusion of everything else. The mind does, however, wander off, but as soon as we realize this we must bring the mind back to the object of meditation. By giving voluntary concentration to a subject, not only are we able to see and think about that subject with greater clarity, but the mind also brings into consciousness all the different ideas and memories associated with the subject. The practical implication is an increased ability to find a solution to any problem. When looking for a solution, we often say "meditate on the problem."

As a deeper state of concentration is developed, the process becomes more intimate and compelling. The mind that holds an idea becomes held by it. Again, this power of the subconscious can be used to build our character. It is known that if we constantly tell ourselves that we are a failure or inferior to others, then eventually we come to believe it. In the same way, if we perceive ourselves to be in possession of a desired trait over and over again, the new image can become a fixed part of our character.

In the mystical tradition, however, the goal of meditation is to narrow down the focus of attention to a point where, eventually, ordinary awareness breaks through to a more intense plane of consciousness. It is a state during which the mind is said to transcend the ordinary plane of awareness and is described as a state where the mind experiences intense joy, happiness, peace, or serenity. It is a state of the greatest silence, or an experience of bliss. In other words, meditation is an experience, a state of being.

There are further practical advantages to meditation. We can function more efficiently, we feel more complete in ourselves, and we are able to realize more of our human potential. We feel closer to ourselves and are better able to relate to others. Our personality structure is strengthened and becomes more integrated. We are able to think and express ourselves with more clarity, and we are more effective in our work and clearer in our goals.

DIFFERENT PATHS TO MEDITATION

Intellectual Path

Just as there are different objects upon which we can meditate, there are different ways in which we can approach meditation (70). The intellectual path appeals to many educated, scientifically oriented, logical, rational individuals. It involves an intellectual understanding of reality. The meditation training further strengthens that understanding.

Whether we accept the meditator's experience of mystical truth or examine the modern physicist's explanation of the world based on the most advanced theories of atomic and subatomic physics, we can come to the same conclusion. Everything that is manifest in the entire universe, both seen and unseen, known and unknown, springs from one source and returns to the same source. Everything is vibrating or shimmering and is in a state of flux or dynamic equilibrium. Everything is permeated with absolute energy or life force. Not only human beings, but every atom of the animal and vegetable kingdom, and every particle of mineral element, is permeated with this absolute energy, although perhaps at different wavelengths. It is not the atom itself but the core and soul of the atom, the field force, which imparts to it direction and the ability to function and is the intelligence of the atom. It makes possible all organic functions, both conscious and subconscious.

Devotional Path

The devotional approach is the one that probably has been practiced more widely until now, particularly in the East. By surrendering to God without hesitation, by loving Him unconditionally, by trusting Him devoutly, and believing that He is present in everything and everyone, the devotee is able to relate to himself and to the universe. He is able to love and care for others, just as he loves and cares for himself. In the face of adversity, whether it is war, famine, or illness in the family, the devotee is able to leave it to God to protect him and his family and can carry on with his routine, feeling secure and at ease. When he firmly believes in the divine presence, when he is satisfied with what has been bestowed upon him in material life, he is not apprehensive or miserable. It is unfortunate that religious fervor has diminished in our society. As a result, it becomes the responsibility of the physician and other health care providers not only to cure our diseases, but also to instill faith and hope in us to face life as well as death. Some meditation schools concentrate on loving ourselves, some on learning to love others, and yet other meditation schools ask us to love God. In the end, they all reach the same point—loving all three and being in complete harmony with the universe.

Physical Path

Another approach is the physical path, in which we learn to become aware of our body and bodily movements. Through hard and long practice, this awareness is heightened to such an extent that it completely fills the field of consciousness to the exclusion of everything else. It also leads to the same result. Hatha Yoga, t'ai chi, the Dervish dances of the Sufi, and their Western equivalent, the Alexander technique of sensory awareness, are some examples. By regularly practicing single-minded concentration on body movements, the meditator gradually strengthens his personality. The different parts of his bodily functions become more integrated with each other, as well as with his personality. A great deal of energy which lies dormant in the body is awakened, and he feels radiant with vitality and life.

Meditation in Action

Finally, there is the approach which involves action. It is also called active meditation or meditation in action. At frequent intervals during the day, if we observe our mind to see what it is doing, it becomes clear that it is busy with wishful thinking, daydreaming, and fantasies of the future. Such useless activity wastes time and energy, and the quality of the work done while daydreaming is poor. By learning to concentrate on an everyday task as if that were the most important thing in the world at that moment, by understanding that each task is only a part of the total harmony with the universe, we come closer to reality. Whenever we are completely engrossed in whatever we are doing, whether as a painter who is painting, a jogger jogging, or a housewife who is simply washing dishes, to the exclusion of everything else in the external world, we are meditating in action. Flower arranging, archery, aikido and karate in the Japanese tradition, and rug weaving in the Sufi (Muslim) tradition are some well-known examples.

COMMITMENT

We should not be fooled into believing that the benefits of meditation can be accomplished by just sitting and repeating some word now and again when we have the time. It is a discipline that requires a lifelong commitment. If we just sit and use the simplest form of meditation like counting our breath for ten to fifteen minutes we will find out soon enough how hard it is to keep our mind concentrated totally and exclusively on this. The first shock and surprise come when we realize how undisciplined our mind really is. It constantly refuses to abide by our will, and the more we try to bring ourselves to the task, the more we find ourselves doing all sorts of things: solving old problems, planning tomorrow's work, and feeling all kinds of sensations and perceptions. Occasionally we get bored or even sleepy. It is important to realize that serious meditation requires perseverance, that it may at times be frustrating, but that it is worth all the effort. Just as muscles cannot be built up with infrequent exercise, neither does enlightenment suddenly appear. It requires a lifelong commitment.

CHOOSING THE RIGHT TECHNIQUE

In the introduction to this chapter it was mentioned that the objects and methods of meditation are many. Because of widespread use and advertisement, many people believe that mantra meditation is the only transcendental meditation. This is not so. All types of meditation, if practiced appropriately and sufficiently, can lead to a state that transcends the limits of ordinary awareness. However, each emphasizes a different quality, and it is important to choose the method with which we feel comfortable, that is, in harmony with our interests and personality, and which flows along with our natural inclination.

Sometimes we need to work with more than one method. If we learn one or more methods, these can be integrated later according to our needs. However, a meditation instructor or institute that expects or requires us to take a vow to remain loyal and attached to them forever or to keep the method they teach a secret or tells us that it is the best is best avoided; if they need a pledge from clients, then they cannot liberate them, and liberation is the ultimate goal of meditation. Changing from one method to another is not a weakness; neither is staying with the first method if we feel it is the right one for us. We should be guided by our inner feelings. However, we should give the method a reasonable trial before abandoning it as unsuitable.

Simple Meditation on Breathing

One simple exercise for bringing awareness to a single subject is concentration on breathing. After you have regulated your breathing and relaxed your body as described, in either a sitting or a reclining position with your eyes closed, you should fix attention on your breath as it enters and leaves your nostrils. The entire focus should be on the nostrils, noting the full passage of each inhalation and exhalation from the beginning to the end. You should feel the sensations of the air going in and out. These sensations may change from that of a dull feather, to itching, to intense pressure, to countless other feelings. There is no right or wrong way. You should simply be aware of your breathing and keep your attention on it. If you have difficulty in keeping your focus fixed, you might try counting 1 on inhalation and 2 on exhalation. If your mind still wanders off, you should just bring it back without feeling agitated.

Mantra Meditation

A neutral word, the name of God, or a verse from a hymn or a prayer is known as a mantra. When it is repeated over and over again, it is an effective way of concentrating the mind.

In Yoga, certain Sanskrit words with the syllables *M*, *H*, and *N* qualify as mantras, such as *Ram* or *Shyam*, which are names of God. My personal mantra is *Swami Narayan*. *Aum* or *Om* is considered to be the basic sound, or the basis of everything. According to the ancient scripture, "All that is past, present, and future is truly Om." All that is beyond this conception of time is also Om. Tibetan lamas and Buddhists from China, Japan, and Indonesia interpret *Om* similarly. An instrument called a *tonoscope*, which can be used to visualize sound in three dimensions, shows that the letter *O* spoken into a microphone produces a perfectly spherical pattern. Thus, *Om* has an interesting significance. It is also worth noting that Christians and Jews say *Amen* and Muslims *Amin* at the end of their prayers. The mantra could be a short phrase (e.g., "Lord Jesus Christ, have mercy on me"). Healing prayers rely on such repetitive sounds for their fundamental effect. However, it is not necessary to have a mantra with religious connotations. You can just repeat a simple neutral word, such as *relaxed* or *one* or *harmony*, or a phrase like "Every day in every way I am getting better and better."

The idea is to set up one thought, one wave, that is repeated over and over again. All you should be consciously thinking of is the mantra. In this way, you become intimate with the sound of the mantra and begin to surrender to or merge into it. The mind will wander off and distracting thoughts will come, but you should not get frustrated and say, "This is hopeless" or "It won't work with me." You should not be disturbed by doubts, discomforts, boredom, or apparent failures but should learn to watch them instead.

The mantra is often practiced along with fingering the beads of a rosary because this helps to keep the attention fixed. As soon as the mind wanders off, the activity of the hand, or the touch of a bead, reminds you of the mantra. The rhythm becomes more compelling as the body works in harmony with the mind. With practice, you may notice that the quality of the mantra changes. When the mind is calm, the mantra will feel subtle and delicate. When the mind is agitated, the mantra will feel strong and coarse. Whatever happens, you should just keep repeating the mantra until the mind becomes more still.

The power of sound waves will be apparent when we consider how modern technology has been able to harness high-frequency sound waves in diagnostic and therapeutic ultrasonic machines. Sound-wave therapy uses as its basic principle the fact that each cell or tissue in the body has its own vibrating frequency, which may be modified by sound waves. Plants seem to grow better when exposed to music than when exposed to random everyday noise. Of course, sound waves can have both good and bad effects. They may make you feel calm or they may make you feel like dancing or tapping, and they may even make you feel wound up and agitated. Hence, care is required in choosing a mantra.

Meditation on Nature

Nature is the easiest object of contemplation. Both therapists and patients can devise meditations in which the patients draw their surroundings into their being through their senses, until they are led into a quiet and peaceful state.

The following suggestions might give you some ideas:

- Visit a meadow, sit under a tree, and just look at the beautiful green fields.
- After you have mown the lawn, savor the smell of freshly cut grass.
- Listen to the music of the ocean or a waterfall. Just forget yourself while you continue to listen. Let the intensity of the sound fill your mind.
- Keep watching the shadow of a boat while you row. See how it shortens or lengthens depending on the situation of the sun. See how the shape changes with the waves as it moves up and down.

- Hold an apple in your hand. Feel its shape and texture, examine its color in detail—smell it. Then close your eyes and just capture all you have seen and felt.
- Taste the wind. What does it carry? Salt from the sea perhaps, or the clean essence of pines from faraway mountains?
- Lie on sun-drenched golden sands and relax until you feel completely limp, as if you are a rag doll with no tension at all.
- Watch the raindrops falling on the ground. Try to see a rainbow in each drop.
- While you are washing the dishes, look at the many colors of the suds. Feel them caressing your fingers. Give your complete attention to the act of washing the dishes.

MEDITATION ESSENTIALS

- Meditate where the distraction of noise, movement, light, and activity of other people are within tolerance level. You may wish to take the telephone off the hook. Some people are more tolerant than others.
- Ensure physical and mental comfort. Make sure that the room is warm. Wear loose clothes. Empty bladder and bowel. Do not practice for at least two hours after a meal. It is most beneficial if you practice twice a day, six hours apart, for example, in the morning before breakfast and again before supper, for about fifteen to twenty minutes each time.
- Adopt a poised posture. In the Eastern tradition, classical lotus, half-lotus, or crossed-legged postures are used, but they are not essential. The Japanese tend to use the thunderbolt posture. You may simply sit in an upright chair. It is essential to have a straight back with-

out rigidity, a comfortable body, and stillness. Your ears should be in line with your shoulders and the tip of your nose in line with your navel. The eyes are kept closed. In Zen, eyes are partially closed gazing at a spot on the floor a few feet ahead. The body should be relaxed, as described under deep muscle relaxation.

- Breathe through your nostrils and down into your abdomen. Make sure that your breathing is regular, slow, and rhythmical.
- Dwell single-mindedly on an object of meditation. The meditation object can be physical, like a fruit, a flower vase, a candle, or a mandala, or a word or phrase repeated mentally or aloud, or a body rhythm like breathing. Count your breath on exhalation from 1 to 10 and start again. Try several methods until you find one which is right for you.
- Passive awareness. This is very important. You must develop a passive and relaxed attitude toward distraction. You will find that thoughts and images will flit in and out of your mind. You will find yourself remembering past images or planning your future. Each time you become conscious that your mind has wandered away (and this will happen many times), just bring it back easily and effortlessly to the object of your meditation. Do this as many times as is necessary, always maintaining the relaxed and passive attitude. As you become more experienced, distracting thoughts and images will lessen. Accept that they are inevitable and maintain an attitude of indifference to them. Meditation is ruined if you keep thinking about meditation: "What is to be done next? What is the experience like? How am I doing? This is no good: I must really try to control my mind." Meditation is nondoing. It is passivity combined with perception. It is pure perception which is formless, wordless, and imageless.

- Regular practice. With practice it becomes easier to still the mind, but you cannot force results.

Meditation is nearly always at least refreshing, relaxing, and peaceful, and for some meditators, on occasion it triggers a peak experience, which is blissful and joyous or even ecstatic.

BENEFITS OF DEEP MUSCLE RELAXATION AND MEDITATION

There is sufficient scientific evidence (8, 101, 140) to show that regular practice of mental and physical relaxation, often known as the relaxation response, leads to the following:

- Reduction in oxygen consumption within minutes by approximately 16 percent. The rate of oxygen consumption reflects the metabolic rate. During six hours of sleep, oxygen consumption gradually falls by 8 to 10 percent. Since we know sleep to be recuperative, we can assume that a few minutes of really deep relaxation can be a quick way of getting recuperation or reenergization of body and mind.
- Reduction in cardiac output, or the amount of blood squeezed through the heart per minute, by over 30 percent during the relaxation response, which reduces the workload of the heart.
- A marked reduction in the level of lactate in the blood during and after the relaxation response. A high concentration of lactate has been known to be associated with anxiety neurosis, panic attacks, and high blood pressure.
- A reduction in sweat gland activity during relaxation, indicating a reduction in the general level of sympathetic activity.

- The respiratory rate is almost halved during relaxation, a reduction indicating a decrease in energy requirement.
- The brainwave pattern becomes more synchronized, a process suggesting coherence between the left and right side of the brain. The waves are also slow and of high amplitude (alpha and theta waves), a condition suggesting relaxation.
- Quicker habituation to noise and adverse stimulation, indicating effective interaction with the environment.
- Increase in alertness and faster reaction time.
- Improved short- and long-term memory.
- Improved academic grades.
- Improved job performance.
- Increased job satisfaction.
- Improved relationships with supervisors.
- Improved relationships with co-workers.
- Reduction in depression.
- Reduction in social inadequacy.
- Increase in self-esteem.
- Reduction in high blood pressure.
- Reduced risk of heart attacks.
- A decrease in tension headaches and migraines.
- Better sleep.
- Improved general health.
- Greater enjoyment of life.
- Better personal and family relationships.
- Improvement in the level of physical energy.
- A better sex life.
- Better concentration at work.

CREATIVE VISUALIZATION

Creative visualization is an adaptation of meditative exercise for specific therapeutic purposes. It is a technique of using our imagination to create what we want in life and is based on the principle that mind and body are intimately connected. Changes in the physical state of our body create changes in our mind and, similarly, every mental image leads to physical changes in the body. We use visual imagery all the time although most of the time we are not conscious of it. Through visualization, we learn to use imagery consciously (39). Images are an important part of our everyday experience. We are equipped with the capacity not just to see what is around us, but to see "with our mind's eye." Images in the mind's eye can be reconstructions of things past, current experiences, or symbolic representations.

Whenever we create something, we always create it in the mind or in thought first. Without thought there is no action. We do not take a bath before we think about or imagine having a bath. An artist first thinks in his mind what the picture may look like before he actually paints it. A dress has be to designed before it can be stitched. When a chef creates a new dish, he imagines in his mind what the new dish will look and taste like before he actually experiments with it. We create what we imagine. It we think of ourselves as beautiful we usually become beautiful because we take care of ourselves and see that we become or remain beautiful.

Images supply us with creative energy or drive. The use and practice of imagery techniques can increase our awareness and understanding of our physical and psychological functioning. Let us do a little exercise. Sit comfortably, close your eyes, relax your body, and imagine you have a lemon in your hand. Now smell it. There is no smell like the smell of a lemon, is there? Now bite the lemon; bite it hard; let all the juices swirl around in your mouth and taste it. What does it taste like? What happened? The saliva just poured into your mouth. Such is the power of your mind. You did not need a real thing. Just imagination created a real physiological response.

Creative visualization can work in two ways. We can either provide ourselves with the opportunity to learn more about previously hidden attitudes and neglected needs, whether physical, psychological, or spiritual, or we can use imagery to influence and direct the functioning of body and mind to gain what we want at the physical, emotional, or spiritual level. For example, you want to get a new job, decorate your bedroom to create a romantic atmosphere, paint a beautiful picture, or write fairy stories (physical levels), or become more assertive, handle a difficult situation with ease, improve your memory and power of concentration, or develop a beautiful relationship (mental levels), or become a radiant being full of love or develop meaningfulness in life (spiritual levels). What you need to do is to get into a relaxed state, conjure up the image of your goal in your mind, and concentrate on the image as long and as frequently as possible; you will be surprised how you can build up a flow of energy which allows you to do the things you need to do to achieve your goal. At first you should set yourself simple tasks. If you can achieve these simple goals, you will find that your confidence gradually increases until you feel nothing is impossible.

Unfortunately, we unconsciously imagine problems, difficulties, obstacles, uncertainties, failures, and limitations, and what we imagine we create for ourselves. When we think ourselves to be ugly we behave in such a way that we become so. When we say to ourselves that it is hopeless, we'll never get enough, or we have to struggle to get our share, we actually make it hopeless or a struggle. When we say to ourselves that love is painful, suffering, and hard work, we behave in such a way that it does turn out to be so. What we are much less aware of is the possibility that through conscious thought and imagination we can achieve what we truly want—love, happy relationships, enjoyment, fulfillment, health, beauty, clarity of expression, and yes, even prosperity and other things our hearts desire (39). As you may be unfamiliar with the skill of consciously visualizing, it may take some time to regain access to and control of this medium. It is likely that images will be discouragingly uncooperative at first, flickering on and off, moving around, and disappearing altogether when inter-rupted by some train of thought.

Visualization is most effective when the mind is quiet, the body relaxed, and the eyes closed. This helps to shut out interference from everyday thoughts and it puts the mind and body in a receptive state. Relaxation also helps to move visualization from seeing in the mind's eye to visualizing "within the body" and furnishes the body with the creative energy or the drive needed to make the wish come true.

As with other therapy, however, we need motivation, understanding, and commitment to be successful. If we are motivated to expand our capacities and increase our personal growth, then creative visualization can truly reveal the miraculous power of the mind, although once we begin to achieve things it may not feel like a miracle anymore. In order to understand how creative visualization works we need to accept that it is more than just wishful thinking. It involves exploring, discovering, and changing our deepest beliefs and most basic attitudes. In the process we may discover how we have been blocking our own goal, how we are preventing ourselves from enjoying life through fear and negative concepts. Once we see these negative attitudes clearly, they can be dissolved, and we thus restore our natural state of happiness and contentment.

It must be borne in mind that we cannot control other people's behavior by this technique, but relaxation at least opens our minds and helps us to become more receptive to others. By doing this we help dissolve barriers and allow others to be more natural.

Four Basic Steps

For creative visualization to be effective you need to follow four basic steps (39):

1. Set a goal that is realistic. To start with, choose goals that are easy to accomplish, before going on to more

difficult or higher goals. Confidence can be built only through success, and setting unrealistic goals is a recipe for a failure and thus negative reinforcement.

2. Create a clear mental picture. It may not be necessary to actually see the image, as long as your thoughts are clear. One person in every ten finds it difficult to make a visual image. Think of your goal in the present tense, as if it already exists, and of yourself within that situation as you desire. This is not cheating yourself but affirming that situations are first created in the mind.

3. Focus on the picture repeatedly, both in a quiet meditative state and also casually during the day whenever you happen to think about it. Make it an integral part of your life. The picture should, however, come to you effortlessly, without striving. Practice before going to sleep or when you wake up in the morning when your body and mind are more relaxed.

4. Give the picture more positive energy as you focus on it, by making positive, encouraging statements or affirmations, as they are often called, and by picturing yourself as actually achieving that goal. During these affirmations suspend all doubts or disbeliefs you may have about achieving your goal.

Dr. Émile Coué, a French chemist and psychotherapist, first coined such positive affirmation in the well-known phrase "Day by day and in every way I am getting better and better." Scientists sometimes laugh at this, but it cured thousands of people with distressing illnesses, including rheumatism, asthma, paralysis of the limbs, stammering, ulcers, and even some tumors. Overnight disappearance of multiple warts through faith healing is a well-known phenomenon. Unfortunately we tend to believe that anything that is so simple can't possibly be good or have powerful or dramatic effect. Jose Silva, the founder and author of the Silva Mind Control Method, suggests that if "you spur your imagination with belief, desire, and expectancy and train to visualize your goals so that you can see, feel, hear, taste, and touch them, you will get what you want" (126).

Examples of Creative Visualization Affirmations

The following are some of the affirmations suggested by Shakti Gawain, the author of *Creative Visualization* (39):

- I am beautiful and lovable.
- I am kind and loving, and I have a great deal to share with others.
- I am talented, intelligent, and creative.
- I have a perfect, satisfying, and well-paid job.
- I love my work, and I am richly rewarded, creatively and financially.
- Everything I need is already within me.
- I love and appreciate myself as I am.
- The more love I have for myself, the more love I have to give others.
- This is a rich universe and there's plenty for all of us.
- I am now full of radiant health and energy.
- I am energetic and full of vitality.
- I am good to my body and my body is good to me.
- I love and accept my body completely.
- I am now ready for all my relationships to work.
- My relationship with _____ is growing happier and more fulfilling every day.

You can make up your own affirmations to suit your needs, and provided they are positive, constructed in the present tense, short and simple, totally right for you, and not directly contradictory to your present feelings and emotions, they should work for you.

12

Developing Communication Skills

The problem of not being able to express our emotions and feelings properly can create stress which need not exist, if only we knew how to communicate properly. Some people have learned early in life that by responding with anger, they can get out of a predicament, while others, whose experience tells them that anger only makes things worse, feel powerless or helpless whenever they are confronted with aggressive people. Lack of assertiveness can create a great deal of internal stress, which, if not expressed, can be buried deeply and can cause hostility or chronic resentment which sometimes explodes as outbursts of anger or weeping. Neither the bottled-up emotion nor the angry outbursts are good for our health, and we need first to understand them and then motivate ourselves to overcome them by developing effective communication skills.

LACK OF ASSERTIVENESS

Sometimes people find it difficult to express their feelings or speak up for their rights. They bottle up emotions for fear of causing unpleasantness or arguments. Lack of assertiveness is a major cause of stress, frustration, and low self-esteem. If you lack assertiveness, people can just bulldoze their way past you by becoming aggressive toward you. Learning to assert yourself also involves raising your self-esteem and feeling good about yourself. By standing up for your rights, you show respect for yourself and will be more likely to win the respect of others. By sacrificing your rights, you encourage others to ill-treat you. You have the right to express yourself so long as you do not violate the rights of others.

As early as 1939, a researcher, Franz Alexander, suggested that more often than not, people who get high blood pressure struggle against their feelings of anger (1). According to him and several subsequent researchers, high-blood-pressure patients have difficulty in expressing themselves. They are unable to speak up for their rights. They resent other people running their lives, making decisions about matters that affect them without consulting them, and setting up rules and regulations about how they should behave, where they should go, and how they should perform their work. These things make them angry but they are unable to express their anger to those who dominate them, so they boil inside, harbor grudges, and sulk, but they don't let others know it. They are afraid that they might cause unpleasant scenes. Nevertheless, they feel infuriated whenever they are criticized in front of others or treated unfairly. This anger and hostility directed inward, often against themselves, can be very destructive. One of William Blake's verses illustrates this point well:

> I was angry with my friend,
> I told my wrath, my wrath did end.
> I was angry with my foe,
> I told it not, my wrath did grow.

More recently a Dutch psychiatrist, J. Groen, listed some of the illnesses that doctors believe are caused by repressed emotions. They include cardiac arrythmia (disturbance of the rhythm of the heartbeats), tachycardia (fast heartbeats), Raynaud's disease (cold and painful fingers which blanch, then turn blue, and finally turn red on exposure to cold), migraine, tension headaches, hyperventilation syndrome, functional diarrhea (diarrhea for which no organic cause is found), habitual constipation, dysmenorrhea (painful periods), premature ejaculation, vaginismus (vaginal spasm), impotence, peptic ulcer, ulcerative colitis, high blood pressure, bronchial asthma, anorexia nervosa, and obesity (45). The assumption, Dr. Groen stated, is that in such cases patients cannot act out their emotions in a simple, direct way, so the internal discharges of the autonomic nervous system are disturbed, and many diseases result. It is from this belief that many doctors and therapists advise their patients to get in touch with their feelings.

Being assertive means that you are able to stand up for yourself, to convey your needs and feelings without misunderstanding, while remaining sympathetic and sensitive to other people's needs and rights (11). It is not becoming insulting or offensive to your friends and relatives or ignoring your spouse and children. Asserting yourself does not involve becoming aggressive, manipulative, or pushy. It should not make people dislike you or the boss fire you. What is called for is not an uncontrolled gush of raw feelings, but a new civility that accommodates the expression of angry emotions.

Assertiveness involves learning to communicate effectively so that, for example, you are not intimidated by the salesperson who is trying to sell you goods you don't want. It means that you can say no to a stranger who is asking you for a date that you are not happy about. It means that you don't give in to unreasonable demands of your employer and you are able to ask pertinent questions of lawyers and doctors courteously and confidently. Assertiveness is an honest expression of your feelings and desires; it is telling people in a firm, open manner where you stand, how you feel, and what your needs are. It is the only way you can have your opinions heard, your claims adjusted, and your rights honored. It also entails taking responsibility for your own actions. Assertive people also recognize that others have exactly the same rights and they listen to others' opinions and claims with respect and talk to them in a tactful manner.

ANGER AND HOSTILITY

Until now it was thought that only anger that is directed inward or anger that is not expressed is harmful and that anger that is directed outward or frankly expressed is all right. This is no longer felt to be true. Frequent outbursts of anger, particularly when they are associated with feelings of hostility, can be very damaging to the health. In fact this is not really a new idea. The fact that anger is damaging goes far back in history. When Rip van Winkle returned home after twenty years of sleep, he found that his ill-tempered wife had long since died of apoplexy. It took a long time for science to realize the truth behind this folk wisdom—that the person who frequently explodes mentally is eventually at risk of exploding physically—for apoplexy is a kind of physical explosion, a bursting of a blood vessel in the brain precipitating a stroke which is often fatal. More and more doctors now believe that anger, hostility, and aggression are important factors affecting health. These factors have also been implicated in the development of high blood pressure and coronary heart disease.

Anger is an emotional state and includes feelings ranging from irritation and annoyance to fury and rage. Such arousal heightens the activity of the sympathetic nervous system and leads to physiological symptoms of stress, such as a rise in blood pressure. Once we calm down, the symptoms subside, unless the arousal is repeated frequently over the minor irritations of life. Occasional angry outbursts when people treat us unkindly or things go wrong for no fault of our own is not a bad thing and may even provide the creative energy to take active measures to prevent ill treatment and gain control over our environment.

Hostility, although it includes angry feelings, is a much broader emotional complex and has connotations of negative, destructive attitudes like hatred, resentment, or animosity. It is more chronic and far more likely to do harm. Research shows that people who harbor grudges or display hostility are more than twice as likely than others to have premature heart attacks (4, 124). Reducing the feeling of hostility requires forgiving. To prevent hostility developing, we learn to manage people effectively.

Causes and Reactions of Anger

Anger does not come in isolation but is associated with other emotions, behaviors, and physical reactions and can be displayed in a variety of ways (133). When the person against whom we wish to show anger is in a dominating position, the anger is often expressed indirectly, as when a wife smashes a cup or kicks the cat, or a husband takes it out on the secretary, or the secretary slams the door. Anger can be expressed directly, particularly by those who are in a dominating position. They can shout, make threats, hurl insults, or strike a blow. Sometimes it is expressed in a more subtle way, like criticizing or making sarcastic remarks or cracking hostile jokes or uttering a jeering laugh. All are aimed at hurting those who made us angry in the first place.

Back in 1894 a psychologist, G. Stanley Hall (48), collected detailed information from questionnaires given to 2,184 people inquiring about situations which made them really angry and how they felt during those angry episodes. The answers varied tremendously. Responses included "I have found it not altogether an unpleasant sensation to be in great rage"; "I am often frightened that I can get so angry and often have a nervous headache later." Some felt different reactions at different times:

"When angry, I feel all of a sudden burning hot, stifled and compelled to make a noise, sometimes I grow icy cold and feel as if I was all blanc mange inside. This feeling is worse than the heat for I seem to be a stone." Others reported that anger produced cardiac sensations, headaches, nose bleeds, mottling on the face, dizziness, tears, snarls, or a complete inability to vocalize. Some would angrily break pens that would not write, throw brushes and pencils that did not work well, tear clothes, smash mirrors, break slates, crush papers, destroy toys, or throw knives, shoes, or books. One woman described in great detail the things which made her angry:

> "The chief causes are contradictions, especially if I am right; slights, especially to my parents or friends, even more than myself; to have my veracity questioned; the sight of my older brother smoking when we are poor; injustice, dislike or hate from those who fear to speak right out; being tired and out of sorts, etc. In the latter mood the least things (will make me angry), like finding books out of place—stupidity in people who will not understand—these make me feel, as a cat must, when stroked the wrong way."

Others felt irritated by thumb rings, bangs, frizzes, short hair on a woman, a hat on one side, baldness, too much style or jewelry, single eyeglasses, flashy ties, heavy watch chains, or many rings.

One woman in my stress management classes said as recently as 1988 that what really made her angry was the fact that men no longer got up and offered their seats to ladies in buses or trains. Thus not only do mental perceptions of insults vary but so do the physical, emotional, and behavioral reactions to anger.

Some people use anger to maintain control over their environment. When anger is unsuccessful in averting danger or removing obstacles, these people feel helpless, in which case the anger is replaced by hopelessness or depression. Whichever way we display anger or irritation, it is like a boomerang; it turns full circle and hits the victim least intended, the one who is angry.

What we need to learn is to manage our anger more effectively, to have control over it rather than to contain it, and to resolve it constructively rather than have explosive outbursts. One of the ways we can do this is by learning effective communication skills.

STRATEGIES FOR IMPROVING ASSERTIVENESS

Identify Problem Areas

The first step in learning to assert yourself is to identify areas where you feel dependent, awkward, uncomfortable, and least confident (11). The situation may occur at home, where others decide what to eat, where to eat, where to go on vacation, or how to spend the money. They may leave dirty dishes in the sink or clothes on the floor, hoping that someone else (you) will see to them. You are expected to adjust to other people's convenience and schedules which are not essential to their work.

The problem may be at work when you find it difficult to ask for a raise in salary or to carry out the personal chores of your boss or to do things you are not employed for, but you are unable to say so. Your colleague in the office may irritate you because instead of discussing mutual problems with you he goes straight to the boss or always lets the phone ring and ring so that eventually you have to answer it. When your patience eventually runs out, one day you shout, "I am sick and tired of you running to the boss directly," or, "For God's sake, answer that telephone; I am not a slave around here."

Do you get angry when someone criticizes you or points out your mistakes? Do you feel guilty if you are occasionally late for work? Do you feel guilty if you want to rearrange your time schedule to suit you? Do you have difficulty in suggesting a better way of working to your superior? Can you say "no" when the boss asks you to do overtime, so that you don't have to break an important date?

The problem may occur in social situations when you find it difficult to return faulty merchandise to the shop, ask your friend not to smoke in your house, or start a conversation with a stranger at a party. List all the problem areas where you would like to be more assertive and then try to tackle these problems, one by one, starting with the easiest and gradually mastering more and more difficult situations.

The second most important step is to have an effective dialogue with yourself. Ask yourself, "What do I want to convey without sounding excessively demanding? How do I make it clear that this is important to me?"

Be Aware of Nonverbal Communication

What we say and how we say it are also part of the continuous process of communication. Even when we say nothing, our silence, gestures, movements, and touch all speak for us. Researchers estimate that more than half the messages people send are conveyed nonverbally (92), and it is important to use our gestures appropriately. Remember the following.

- Making eye-to-eye contact is necessary to convey that you are listening.
- Yawning or closing your eyes may give the impression that you are not interested.
- Simultaneously raising the eyebrows and frowning may mean that you are doubtful.
- Standing may be more intimidating than sitting.

- A firm voice indicates that you are serious and is particularly effective if you get the impression that the person you are talking to is taking your words too lightly.
- A lively intonation of voice conveys ease and stops you from sounding intimidating.
- Excessive use of "um" and "ah" shows uncertainty.
- To show that you are sincere, you must avoid unnecessary gestures, gimmicks, smiles, or lip smacking.
- To convey ease, avoid sitting stiffly, and uncross your arms and legs.

Change Your Dialogue

When talking to someone who has previously dominated you, be polite but firm (avoid apologizing or shouting), use *I* instead of *it*, be direct and to the point, and avoid long explanations. Start off by saying no if you want to refuse a request, and acknowledge others' feelings. Speak in a clear voice to get your message across. For example, you can tell your spouse, "I don't want to go to an Indian restaurant today. I would like to go to a Chinese one today," rather than, "You always pick an Indian restaurant. I am sick and tired of Indian food," or say nothing and endure. You can tell your children or spouse, "I don't like dirty dishes lying around in the sink. Will you please wash your dishes before you leave the kitchen?" rather than, "How dare you leave dishes in the sink. Do you think I am your slave?" or just washing them yourself to keep peace and quiet. You can express your desire for a different vacation by saying, "I would like to go to some historic place this year," rather than reluctantly and silently putting up with a regular seaside vacation or remarking, "Why don't you pick something more intellectual rather than a boring seaside vacation every year?"

To your colleague you may say, "I don't like answering the phone all the time for you, so you can answer the next call," or "I would like you to discuss our mutual problem with me first, before you take it to the boss." You can tell your boss, "I would like to help but I can't do any overtime today because I have an important engagement," or "I am more than willing to do things I am employed to do, but shopping for your wife isn't one of them."

I would like to remind you, though, that things are not always as simple as they sound, and if you are not careful, you may sound as though you are making a demand or being rude, and that will only make things worse. Some researchers say that direct confrontations may themselves produce anxiety and carry a certain risk of their own. Dr. Ernest Harburg and his colleagues studied a random sample of men and women living in Detroit. The majority of working-class men said that they would report an unjust boss to the union or to someone higher up, or that they would protest to him directly. Unfortunately, people who would use this kind of strategy of expressing anger toward their boss showed the highest blood pressure. This was specifically true of young black men who were living in stressful neighborhoods with high rates of crime, divorce, and unemployment. People who showed the lowest blood pressure turned out to be those who would just walk away from a belligerent boss and let the storm blow over or who would try to reason with him (49).

The same investigators, however, found that being angry with prejudiced homeowners (landlords) or an explosive police officer was appropriate because the group with such a belief also had lower blood pressure compared with those who would keep quiet about their anger or who would feel guilty about expressing it! The best strategy for handling anger is neither to suppress it nor to confront it aggressively, but to wait until both you and the person who has insulted you have calmed down, then to reflect on the matter, and finally to try to reason with him.

Be Persistent

The first thing to learn in being assertive is persistence (129). You usually lose in a conflict because you give up too easily. The important lesson in being assertive is to keep saying what you want over and over again, in the same tone of voice. People will try to put you off or say things that will anger you, or they will try other strategies to get you off their back, but you should neither become angry nor budge an inch until you get a satisfactory answer.

For example, you buy six bath towels at a department store, but when you check at home, you find only five in the bag. You go back to the store, see the same assistant, tell her that you were short of one towel, and say, "I want my towel." She will probably tell you, "Maybe you dropped it somewhere, in your car or in a bus." You say, "No, I haven't; I want my towel." She then tells you she hasn't got the authority to give you the missing towel. You ask to see the manager and repeat, "I want my towel." She tells you to come back again because the manager is too busy today. You insist on seeing the manager and repeat, "I want my towel." Then she tells you to go to the fifth floor, Room X, to see the manager, but you insist that you are not going anywhere and say, "Please call the manager here." Eventually the manager comes, and you repeat that you were given only five towels instead of six and say, "I want my towel." He starts the same arguments, that you may have dropped one in the car or a bus, and you repeat the same things again until he gives you the missing towel.

Sometimes you may not achieve your goal immediately, but the fact that you are exercising your assertive right will make you feel good about yourself, and keeping your self-respect is an important part of being assertive.

Make a Workable Compromise

Whenever you feel that your self-respect is not in question, you can offer an acceptable compromise (129). For example, you could offer to wait for a certain time for a shop to replace defective goods or agree to do what the other person wants, next time. You can always bargain with another person for your material goal if this does not affect your self-respect. However, there are certain exceptions, like legal or physical matters. It would be futile to persist in this "broken record" style of dialogue with an angry judge or an unreasonable police officer, although this doesn't mean you have to swallow your pride. If you believe in your case, you have the option of going to a higher court or of complaining in writing about the police officer to his superior. Another situation where assertiveness would be foolish is when you are confronting violence. It would be better to comply with someone who is pointing a gun at you.

Assertive Social Conversation

Assertive behavior is much more than demanding your rights from other people or preventing other people from manipulating you. Being in a social environment means communicating with another person about who you are, what you do, what your interests are, or what you expect out of life. If the other person is equally assertive, this type of communication can form a basis for a mutually rewarding, self-sustaining relationship. It also helps you to stop a dead-end relationship because you find out early that there are no common interests and therefore you stop wasting your time. In order to become an assertive communicator in a social setting, you must first learn to listen to other people and to follow up on information freely given to you. If you do this you are assertively prompting and making it easier for them to continue talking because of your interest. Second, you must disclose information about yourself so that social communication flows both ways. Without this self-disclosure the other person may feel that you are simply prying into his personal life without sharing yours.

Understand Your Critic

We often get hurt by other people's negative criticism. The lower we hold ourselves in our esteem, the more sensitive or touchy we become, and the more touchy we are, the more the criticism is likely to deflate our self-esteem. In actual fact criticism cannot affect real self-esteem, which is innate and independent of others' opinions, but if we lack self-esteem, people can rub us up the wrong way and make us defensive or, according to Matthew McKay and Patrick Fanning, make us respond in one of three undesirable ways: too aggressively, too passively, or passive-aggressively (76).

When you respond aggressively you immediately mount a counterattack. The possible advantage is that it may get the critic off your back, for the time being. But sooner or later he will be back with bigger and bigger ammunition until the episode escalates into a bitter war. Your aggressive style of responding will do nothing to boost your self-esteem and it will prevent you from building a deeper friendship with others.

If you are too passive, you may quickly feel intimidated by others' criticism and immediately agree or apologize. Since the critic can't pick a fight with you anymore he will leave you alone but you will certainly feel sorry for yourself for not having stood up for yourself and your self-esteem will have taken a further knock.

Then there is a passive-aggressive style of responding to criticism; you apologize or agree instantly but are left seething inside, and later you will consciously or unconsciously try to get even by subversive or indirect means. This has the effect of lowering your self-esteem twice—first when you apologize and again when you try to attack covertly. Eventually you end up hating yourself.

Before you can respond in a healthier, assertive way, you need to understand why the critic has developed such an irritating style of communication. His powerful needs, his ingrained beliefs, his current emotional and biological states, his innate constitution and his habitual patterns of behavior all contribute to his mode of communicating.

Respond to Your Critic Appropriately

Once you understand your critic, it becomes easier to adopt a less defensive and more assertive way of responding, in which you neither attack nor surrender to the critic. You don't even have to resort to subversion but you directly and frankly assert yourself and clear up misunderstandings. Again, according to McKay and Fanning, you can choose one of the three techniques that is appropriate for the circumstances: acknowledge but don't apologize, accept in principle, or ask for clarification (76).

Acknowledge But Don't Apologize. In the first technique you acknowledge what you consider was accurate in the criticism and ignore the rest. For example, you say the critic is right; even paraphrase his words so the critic thinks you are sincere. But there is no need to apologize. Saying things like "You are right. I should have done it that way. Thanks for reminding me" immediately disarms the critic without wounding your self-esteem. However, this technique works only when there is truth in what the critic is saying, even though his style of communication is abhorrent. Therefore, if you don't think his criticism is accurate in substance, you can use the second technique of token agreement.

Agree in Principle. When the critic is inaccurate and unconstructive, the best you can do is to agree in part, in probability, or in principle, by saying, "Yes, you may possibly be right," or "I may have made a mistake here." You may agree with his logic but not his assessment. This way you can silence your critic without sacrificing your sense of self-worth.

Ask for Clarification. A lot of criticism is vague. People often use emotionally loaded words which do not specify the problem and you are not sure what the critic is trying to say or what wrong you have done. The way to take the heat out of the matter is to ask probing questions until you are clear in your mind about the substance of the criticism. Ask questions like "What offended you?"; "How did I let you down?"; "Why do you think so?"; and "What exactly do you want me to do?" Asking questions like these in an inquisitive and nonargumentative tone of voice will calm your critic and clarify the problem. Once you have got all the information you want you will know whether to acknowledge the criticism or just agree in probability.

STRATEGIES FOR MANAGING ANGER

Respond Positively to Criticism

If people criticize you, remember that you must be important enough for people to get satisfaction out of it. Why do you think that Kitty Kelly wrote an entire book to expose points of Nancy Reagan? Would people be interested in reading about an ordinary housewife who may be having an affair or may be dominating her husband? Not at all. There is a saying that "No one kicks a dead dog."

There will be times when you will be criticized whatever you do: damned if you do, damned if you don't. Do what you think is right and ignore the unjust criticism. It is not possible to please everyone. Abraham Lincoln once said that all you can do is your best about handling criticism of others, and Winston Churchill had this literary gem framed and hung in his study at Chartwell:

> If I were to try to read, much less to answer all the attacks made on me, this shop might as well be closed for any other business. I do the best I know how—the very best I can; and I mean to keep on doing so until the end. If the end brings me out all right, then what is said against me won't matter. If the end brings me out wrong, the ten angels swearing I was right would make no difference.

Help Anger Simmer Down

Anger does not occur in isolation. It is part and parcel of the arousal response, which involves both the body and the mind. You cannot be angry in the mind and completely relaxed in the body; neither are you completely at the mercy of unconscious emotional forces, because of your ability to think and choose how you interpret situations or to act. Feelings of anxiety make you either compliant or aggressive. You can't be assertive if you are uptight. All your energy is spent in being tense and anxious. Therefore it is vital to relax and compose yourself. In addition you can use incompatible behavior or emergency stop techniques. By choosing incompatible behavior or an emergency stop, you can learn to control anger or explosive outbursts. Ethel Roskies suggests that: whenever you recognize yourself shouting, talk slowly. You can't talk slowly and shout at the same time (115). By deliberately talking slowly, you control your anger. Another technique is to use an emergency stop. You can decide in advance an appropriate behavior, which you will use as soon as you recognize that you are becoming angry. For example, you can decide (and then make a habit of practicing it) that as soon as you hear yourself shouting, you will cross your fingers, take one deep breath, and count to 5 before you start talking again. The classic advice of counting to 10 or its variations has survived for centuries:

> When angry, count ten before you speak; if very angry, an hundred.
> THOMAS JEFFERSON
> When angry, count four, when very angry, swear.
> MARK TWAIN

Swearing, however, is likely to fuel the flame. Here I think Plutarch made the most pertinent observations when he said:

> For he who gives no fuel to fire puts it out, and likewise he who does not in the beginning nurse his wrath and does not puff himself up with anger, takes precautions against it and destroys it.

Another way to take the heat out of anger is to plot a revenge in as much detail as possible on a piece of paper or with a therapist. This strategy was shared by a therapist who took one of my training classes. He suggested that a quick murder was out because we want an enemy to suffer. This theoretical revenge plotting gets so ridiculous that we eventually laugh at it, and anger is automatically dissolved.

Use Anger Creatively

Anger is a sudden release of energy. Some are more inclined to have this outburst of energy than others. However, how you use this energy often depends on your personality. It is possible, however, to channel this energy more creatively. A psychologist, Alan Sroufe (131), once put it this way:

> A child who has a rapid tempo may be seething with anger, hostile to other children, unable to control his or her

impulses, and filled with feelings of worthlessness. But a child who has a rapid tempo also may be eager, spirited, effective and a pleasure to others and may like him or herself.

The fact that anger can be used creatively is explicit in the following remarks:

> When I am angry, I can write, pray, and preach well, for then my whole temperament is quickened, my understanding sharpened and all mundane vexations and temptations gone.
>
> MARTIN LUTHER

Catharsis

Some therapists believe that one should use any form of aggressive release of anger that comes to mind, instead of harboring grudges. This release may be shouting, screaming, biting, kicking, slapping, or any other form of verbal or physical assault. Unfortunately this "getting in touch with" our feelings does not always exorcise anger and often inflames it. The tendency to become irritated, angry, or furious over the trivial errors of others ruins our relationships with business or professional associates and members of our family. During anger, stress hormones known as *epinephrine* and norepinephrine are released. If we allow our aggressive behavior to become permissible, there is a danger that we may become addicted to stress hormones.

We cannot change people's behavior by angry words or nasty criticisms. The way to get the best out of people is through appreciation and encouragement. A research study showed that the most important factor related to why wives leave their husbands was "lack of appreciation." Criticism puts people on the defensive and makes them strive to justify themselves. It hurts people's pride, wounds their sense of importance, and arouses their resentment. Dale Carnegie, the author of the best-selling book *How to Win Friends and Influence People* (19), stated "When dealing with people, let us remember that we are not dealing with creatures of logic. We are dealing with creatures of emotion, creatures bristling with prejudice and motivated by pride and vanity." The best way to criticize people is to call their attention to their failings indirectly.

Learn the Art of Forgiving

We all, at some time or other, have been deeply hurt, knowingly or unknowingly, by someone in our life. If that person happens to be a person we love, whether parent, lover, spouse, child, or a friend we trusted and cared about, the hurt is likely to be deep. If we feel the treatment we were given was completely unfair or undeserved, it may continue to fester and leave us with a permanent scar unless we find it in our heart to forgive. Fortunately love's power to forgive is stronger than hate's power to take revenge (128).

We are not talking about the trivial mistakes or irritations frequently caused by people, which can be forgotten in time. We are talking about the insufferable pain when we feel outraged by the way we are lowered beneath human dignity—pain so deep that we may even wonder why we should forgive. We may even ask, "Wouldn't it encourage people to commit the same hurtful act again?" The answer is that we need to forgive them for our own sake. It is the only way to bring fairness into this unfair world. When we forgive, we do ourselves a great service because if we don't forgive, our wound can turn into hate and hate can kill.

When someone close to us shows disloyalty or commits an act of brutality or betrayal, we can become hateful. We may even secretly wish that lightning might strike that person down. It would, at least, be difficult to wish him success. Such hate needs healing and forgiveness for our own good since, without forgiveness, it would hurt us more than the person we hate. We may try to suppress hate because we want to believe that we are too nice to harbor malice. Unfortunately, such a denial doesn't cure us of the hostility which can then travel under the surface and may later explode as an angry outburst.

How to Forgive. The following suggestions are based on advice given by Lewis Smedes, the author of *Forget and Forgive* (128):

- To begin with, you need to separate the person from the hurt he has caused. View him as a weak, needy, not infallible human being and then set him free. If you find yourself wishing him good luck (which may be days or years later), you are well on your way to forgiving him.
- You then tell him you forgive him. Do this without any strings attached. Forgiving is not easy, but you need it for your own healing and peace of mind more than the person who has hurt you, and who may or may not care about your forgiveness. There is no reason why you should suffer. So just forgive and be free. Tell him, "What you did was bad, but I forgive you."
- However, forgiving doesn't mean losing your dignity. It doesn't mean that you restore the person to his previous place in your life, unless he regrets his actions and asks for your forgiveness. If that does not happen you will have to settle for your own healing and forgive the person without allowing him the same place back in your life.
- Be patient. The hate habit is hard to break. Forgiving may take several attempts and a long period of time. Sometimes it is so slow that you don't actually know when you finally forgave.

- It is easier to forgive if you can understand what's going on in the mind of the person who betrayed you. It may be inferiority, ignorance, false pride, or a need for recognition. Smugness or cruelty may be his way of coping with the problem. You need to understand that even those you love dearly have their own unique personality and affliction. You cannot expect other people, or even your own children, to be made in your image. You can be tolerant of their affliction, even pity them for having it, but you have to accept them for what they are. It is also necessary to reflect on your own behavior. The fault may lie within your own shortcomings or insecurity; after all, you, too, are human.
- Forgiving doesn't mean that you will never feel angry about the event that hurt you. It may still happen; but forgiving takes the passion out of hate. The malice no longer exists.
- Forgiving is the only way to be fair to yourself. You may feel that it is unfair to forgive a person who is unfair to you. But what is the alternative? Revenge? An eye for an eye? A tooth for a tooth? Unfortunately, trying to take revenge may escalate and finally perpetuate unfairness, because your measurement of the hurt and the degree of the revenge are bound to differ from the measurement of the person who committed the evil deed in the first place. Trying to get even is like playing a loser's game, adding flame to the fire and leading eventually to self-destruction. How rightly Gandhi said that if we insist on an "eye for an eye, the whole world will be blind." Besides, you may be too old and weak to take revenge, or those who hurt you may now be dead or a long way away. By not forgiving, you condemn yourself to lifelong torment.
- Hate is powerful and you may feel more macho telling someone, "Get the hell out of here," than saying "I forgive you." But look at it this way. Who wins the game?

The person who penetrates your heart with his sharp words or awful deeds and then goes about his own business as if nothing has happened, or you who are left behind suffering?

- Sometimes we use hate as a mask to hide our own weakness. Hating is easier than admitting our fault or weakness. Putting other people down can cover up our human frailties. After all, there is no such thing as a totally good person and a totally bad person. If we look at the picture as a whole, it is difficult to define things only in terms of black and white. We might not be quite such innocents as we think we are. Once we admit to ourselves that we, too, are human beings, and that there is no reason to be ashamed of a single human error, it becomes unnecessary to use the disguise of hate.

- Forgiving requires courage and strength to face up to reality. In order to avoid the dilemma of forgiving, we sometimes do not acknowledge the crime. Self-deception is easier than having to forgive the person we love. Yet forgiving doesn't mean covering up for people we love. The only way they can gain self-respect is to be accountable for their own deeds.

- Don't judge the person who has betrayed your trust. Instead, put yourself in his shoes and ask; "If I had been in his place, subject to the same influences and circumstances he was exposed to, might I have done the same thing?" Someday you may need to be forgiven. Would you have the right to expect forgiveness of others if you refuse to forgive someone today for his thoughtless deed?

13

Other Strategies for Managing Stress

BE AWARE

Recognizing the problem is half the battle. Without knowing what stress is, and how it may strain our health, we will not be able to recognize it. Awareness is of primary importance if we are to learn to manage stress effectively. Our body is often the first place to reveal signs of a problem. Unfortunately, our upbringing often trains us to be stoic, and in our anxiety not to appear weak, we often deny signs of stress. This is particularly true of many men.

We have already discussed the mental, emotional, physical, and behavioral signs of stress, as well as possible occupational, domestic, social, political, and economic stressors and the contexts in which they are likely to produce stress. Remember that your vulnerability is continuously changing. Your susceptibility is affected by your personality attributes: the number of life changes requiring adaptation which have occurred in the recent past, as well as your general health, nutritional state, physical fitness, age, and previous training or experience. There are times when your resistance is so low that even a minor irritation seems a major provocation. At other times, you feel ready to tackle even a major obstacle with ease and confidence.

Get into the habit of mentally noting daily stressors and their effects. If necessary keep a stress diary in which you write down, every hour, what you are doing and if you have any stress symptoms, whether physical, emotional, mental, or behavioral.

AVOID UNNECESSARY STRESS

You don't have to try to avoid all stress, even if that were possible. The human performance curve shows that performance improves with a certain amount of arousal or effort. Too little stress can be as frustrating and stressful as too much stress. Optimum stress provides a creative challenge. Know your limits and recognize the signs of overloading, like tiredness and irritation, and then accept them as signals for a little break. Try to avoid the most explosive situations or continuing perseverance with your efforts to the point of exhaustion. The key word, as in all things, is *balance*. If maximum stress is given ten points and minimal stress is given one point, you should try to maintain a level of five to six points.

ANTICIPATE STRESS AND BE PREPARED

The best time to avoid mistakes is before they happen. How you anticipate events affects your response. If you are fearful about an event, the body will respond as if you are actually experiencing the event with fright. If, on the other hand, you think you will be able to handle the situation, your mind and body will remain relaxed. Knowing how your body responds to mental images, you can prepare yourself mentally to face the future situation.

Sometimes the situation is quite obvious. For example, making an important presentation or the arrival of a new boss may create uncertainty, resulting in mental or physical tension. At other times you are unaware of the situation. All you know is that you just don't feel comfortable. Keeping a stress diary may help you to identify possible stressors. Once you know the problem, you can make plans to deal with it.

Strategies for Positive Anticipation

Imagine the Forthcoming Event. Identify situations which previously left you tense or uncomfortable. Consider what specific part of that situation was stressful. Don't dwell on the faulty behavior of a particular person, but on how that person affected you.

Prepare Adequately. There is no substitute for adequate preparation. Inadequate preparation leads to unnecessary anxiety. Specify your goals and work out all the details. If it is your reaction to hostile remarks which is likely to be stressful, prepare in advance for ways of dealing with those remarks without getting upset.

Rehearse the Night Before. Imagine the situation. Imagine yourself performing the task in detail with confidence. Continue practicing this image until you feel comfortable. Tell yourself that if you hear hostile remarks you are going to take a deep breath, and that in a slow, calm voice you are going to focus only on the business in hand.

Plan Some Pleasurable Activity. If the tension is getting to an uncomfortable level during your preparation time, take a break to go for a walk or swim or participate in some other sporting activity you like. Stretch your body, snap your fingers, have a big yawn. All these activities discharge nervous energy and prevent tension from mounting up.

Prepare for the Worst. Imagine the worst that can happen and how you would cope with it. If there is no constructive way in which you can confront the situation, think about how you can withdraw from the situation without losing face.

On the Day of the Stressful Event. When you get out of bed, imagine getting through your day comfortably. Keep focusing on how you will deal with the situation calmly and deliberately.

Relax Before the Event. Just before the event, take a few slow deep breaths, relax your shoulders, unclench your jaw and fists, uncross your legs, and allow the body to relax.

Expect Some Stress. Some stress is necessary to improve your performance, so don't expect to wipe it out completely. In addition, changing long-standing habits is not easy and success cannot be expected every time, despite all the hard work you have done. Develop an attitude of "Win some, lose some."

Take Time Out to Recuperate. As soon as the stressful event is over take time off to recuperate. Plan some pleasurable activity. If tension has accumulated, release it through vigorous activity. Alternatively, curl up with a good book.

Reward Yourself. Make sure you give yourself credit for a job well done. Even if you did not completely master the situation, whatever success you did have is a praiseworthy achievement and deserves compliments. Do something more tangible. Have your hair done, pamper yourself with a massage, buy yourself a book or record, or go to that gourmet restaurant for a good dinner.

Anticipating Regular Events

When we think of stress, we have a tendency to think of it in terms of sudden and unexpected happenings in our life. In fact, most of our stress comes from regular recurrences of the same old problems: preparing for a weekly meeting with hostile co-workers; trying to finish paperwork the night before a deadline; lining up at the post office every Friday. By learning to recognize and prepare for these recurrent problems, we can achieve better control over them. We can consciously take one of several options:

- Avoiding those situations
- Taking effective preventive action
- Being prepared to confront the situation head-on
- Reevaluating our strategy periodically

Sometimes people feel that anticipation is unnatural or unnecessary, but successful troubleshooting requires anticipating problems so that the appropriate action can be taken. After you have been engaged in positive anticipation for a while, reevaluate the situation. Have you been successful in achieving your goal? Can you improve your strategy? Would changing your strategy be more beneficial?

STRESS IS NOT BLACK AND WHITE

We discussed earlier how stress is associated not only with physical tension or maladaptive behavior, but also with automatic thoughts and feelings. Often we are unaware of them. When we do consciously catch them, however, we consider them absolute truths or irrevocable facts: they provide an interpretation of events and predictions about a situation. The last time you were really stressed or upset, do you remember thinking one of the following?

- I can never do anything right.
- I always mess things up.
- It's completely hopeless and futile.
- I can never accept that position.

There is a tendency, when stressed or upset, to view everything in black and white, to generalize or attach undue significance to some selective aspect of that event. Unfortunately, the body reacts according to the way the mind interprets a situation and thus stress can often be magnified or even perpetuated. If we can learn to replace those thoughts of "beyond a reasonable doubt" with more relative terms, for instance, by substituting *often* for *always*, *rarely* for *never*, and *might* for all our *musts* and *shoulds*, we can learn to modulate our stress response. By analyzing our automatic thoughts and translating them into more manageable difficulties, we can avoid becoming overwhelmed, helpless, or out of control. We go to pieces because we imagine the situation to be far more intimidating than it really is.

The experience of many clinicians and the results of research studies suggest that those people who redefine a stressful situation so that it takes on a slightly different and more benign meaning seem both to suffer a less intense physiological response and to recover faster. Next time you feel tense or stressed, follow your thoughts and confront them. See if you can relabel the situation and you may be pleasantly surprised with the results.

Negative Self-Talk and Positive Antidotes

The point is that we do have a choice in how we program ourselves. Negative programming will lead to stress, while positive programming will act as an antidote in times of stress. The following are common negative self-comments and the alternative positive statements:

1. *Negative:* I can't help it if other people or things upset me.
   Positive: I can choose how I react. It is only I who upsets me.
2. *Negative:* I have no control over the nature or severity of my feelings, or how long those feelings last.
   Positive: I may not be able to control getting upset, but I have considerable control over how deeply I feel and how long my emotional reactions last.
3. *Negative:* It's all genetics. My mother was just like me.
   Positive: Feelings and behaviors are not inherited but learned in childhood. If they are not serving my purpose, I can unlearn them.
4. *Negative:* I can't change the way I react.
   Positive: Through realistic, constructive self-talk I can change the way I react to stressful situations.
5. *Negative:* Things should and must happen the way I want them to.
   Positive: It would be great if everything went my way. But that's not always possible and I am prepared to take things as they come.
6. *Negative:* I can't believe this is happening to me. I don't understand it. How can anyone treat me like this when I have tried so hard to please?
   Positive: Well, if I put my mind to it I can understand what's happening to me.

7. *Negative:* It's absolutely terrible; no one could stand it.
   Positive: Things are never as bad as they first seem or as I tend to make them out. I must learn not to blow things out of all proportion.
8. *Negative:* I will never win. I am a born loser.
   Positive: I can accept what I am. Even with certain shortcomings, everything is not lost.
9. *Negative:* I am nobody and nobody really thinks anything of me.
   Positive: Others will accept me the way I present myself and I can certainly present myself better.
10. *Negative:* It's hopeless. Things will never change.
    Positive: There is always hope. Things will look better in the long run, especially if I learn to cope with them better.
11. *Negative:* I am incredibly nervous.
    Positive: I get nervous sometimes, but who doesn't?
12. *Negative:* I get terribly upset.
    Positive: I get rather upset now and again.
13. *Negative:* I am lazy, idle, good for nothing.
    Positive: Sometimes I tend to get lazy, but I can get myself back on track again.
14. *Negative:* I always make mistakes.
    Positive: Everyone makes a mistake once in a while.
15. *Negative:* I always mess things up.
    Positive: Sometimes I spoil things, but so do others.

MASTER PROBLEM-SOLVING SKILLS

Another technique you can use to modulate your stress response is to appraise your stressor or stress response as a problem to be solved. Once you learn to look at it more objectively, you become emotionally detached from your stress, and thus, a vicious circle is broken. The following are steps to be followed in problem-solving training (87, 88):

- Define the stressor or stress response as a problem to be solved. Ask yourself what is the nature of the problem.
- Set realistic goals and state them as clearly as possible. Ask yourself what you want in the end.
- Open your mind to a wide range of possible alternative solutions irrespective of how farfetched or difficult to achieve they may be. List all the possible things you might do, including those which are only remotely possible.
- Imagine how other people might respond if they were asked to deal with similarly stressful situations. If necessary, talk to them.
- Evaluate the pros and cons for each alternative solution in terms of its practicality, the effort involved, and its possible benefits. Rank order them from the least effective to the most effective strategies. Consider the consequences. What's the best that can happen? What's the worst that can happen?
- Visualize those strategies in your mind and rehearse them in graduated steps. Decide on the most feasible and acceptable strategy. What is your plan of action?
- Rehearse the decided strategy and put it into practice. Expect some failure. In any new effort, beginning is the hardest part. Give yourself credit for your initial steps.
- Reward yourself for trying. Giving yourself a pat on the back is essential reinforcement for further action.
- Evaluate the result. Reconsider the original problem in the light of the attempt. Did it work? Is modification of the strategy necessary?

Problem-Solving Exercise

What's the problem? _____

_____

What's the goal? _____

_____

Possible alternative solutions:

                                                                           Practicality   *Effort*

1.

2.

3.

4.

5.

6.

7.

How to Rank Order

Extremely easy to implement	1	2	3	4	5	Most difficult to implement
Minimum effort required	1	2	3	4	5	Maximum effort required

MANAGE TIME EFFECTIVELY

"But I don't have time to relax." "I have too many things to do and not enough time to do them in." Do these statements sound familiar to you? Many people feel the same way. In reality, we must cope with life as it is and not as we would like it to be. A lot of unnecessary stress comes because we do not use time wisely. It does not mean slowing ourselves down. What it does mean is utilizing our time more efficiently to carry out the things which are really important. A busy person is not necessarily under stress. Nor does getting rid of stress mean being slow. We must have time to feel a sense of accomplishment. If we are continuously being rushed and pushed, we may get so overwhelmed or confused that we may lose all perspective, become less efficient, and therefore be under greater pressure. It is up to us how we use the twenty-four hours we have been given in a day.

To see how you have been using time in the last three working days, ask yourself:

- Are you completely happy with the way you used your time?
- If not, why not?
- What could you have done to use your time more satisfactorily?

It is important to plan your day as well as to plan the month and the year. You have to spend time to make time. Have a few minutes set aside each day and each week to plan your activities. Managing your time well will reduce stress.

Strategies for Effective Management of Time

Be in control of your time rather than letting time control you. The following are some general tips:

- Plan and organize your timetable well ahead. Record regularly occurring events several weeks or months in advance.
- Allow space between projects. You need time to catch your breath between activities and to recover physically and psychologically.
- Allow at least one-tenth of your time to be "free time" or flextime in order to accommodate unexpected tasks.
- Give priority to those tasks that have to be achieved and allot a larger part of your time to high-priority tasks. Put off any less urgent tasks. It is perfectly all right to put off tasks today that can be done tomorrow.
- Clear your desk of all papers except those which relate to the immediate problems at hand. A desk cluttered with unanswered mail and unfinished reports is a constant reminder of millions of things to do and no time to do them in.
- Inform people of time limits in advance. This way they will not waste your time or expect extra time to complete the task.
- Do routine tasks, like handling paperwork, only once a day and preferably at the same time. Group similar tasks together and you will be surprised by how fast they are completed.
- Intersperse dull jobs with interesting jobs and tiring jobs with easier ones.
- Take the telephone off the hook when you don't want to be disturbed. Somehow, each day you should have time just for yourself.
- Write in your leisure, pleasure, relaxation, and exercise activities as well as your work tasks, as they are essential for recharging your energy for efficient working. Allow time for social and family commitments.
- Try getting up half an hour earlier or reducing your television time. Whatever you do, don't waste time feeling guilty about what you could not do.

- Do one task at a time before going on to the next. People feel less apprehensive if a long line of tasks is kept out of sight. However, don't make a fetish of it. Not all tasks can be completed at one sitting.
- Plan in terms of time rather than tasks. For example, instead of thinking, "I have ten things to do," try thinking, "I have six hours. What can I reasonably do in that time?"
- Take time to sit down and plan your day. List things you want done and then assign high, medium, or low priority to each of them. Start with top-priority jobs.
- Write down things you like to do and things you don't enjoy. Consult your supervisor to see if your work can be structured around the things you enjoy doing.
- Important or big tasks which demand time, energy, and concentration should be done when you are feeling fresh and energetic. Leave small jobs or routine tasks to be done later when you may or may not be in peak condition.
- Don't keep putting off decisions. If you have the necessary facts available, solve the problem then and there. Unresolved problems or unfinished business are a source of tension and worry which dissipate your energy.
- Put aside some time for things you really have been wanting to do but that your daily routine has not allowed you to get down to. Cross those periods out in your diary as not available for routine work, and try to safeguard them.

Delegating Tasks

Many shrewd people know that the secret of getting a lot of things done in the short time available is to get others to do them. In an efficient household, chores are delegated to the spouse as well as the children. People at the top have reached their position because they are good at using this tactic. A competent supervisor knows how to delegate work effectively. You may find the following tips useful:

- Don't always carry the impression that other people can't do the job as well as you. If you give them the opportunity, they will do the tasks just as well.
- It is not necessary to carry out every task to its ultimate perfection.
- You are not indispensable. The world and your company will still go on after you are gone.
- Let people use their own imagination and skill to carry out tasks. Just tell them what end results you expect.
- Telling people in detail how to do a job robs them of their creativity, as they cannot take pride in their achievement when the tasks are carried out under detailed instructions.
- Don't oversupervise. People work better if you are not breathing down their necks.
- Remain in charge. Giving a free hand doesn't mean that you give in to every desire of the people working under you. Don't be afraid to say no if it is necessary.

HAVE HUMOR IN YOUR LIFE

The idea that laughter is the best medicine is not new. It is part of folklore. But like any folk remedy, we are usually skeptical about it, unless there is scientific evidence to back the claim or we have had personal experience of its benefit or know of someone having been helped by it. A true story in which someone laughed his way out of a crippling disease is cited below and it should make us all think that perhaps we should have regular laughs in our life.

Norman Cousins, the author of *Anatomy of an Illness*, narrates his personal experience in his book (24). In 1964 he was crippled with a serious illness affecting all his joints and muscles. Doctors diagnosed it as connective tissue disorder, wherein his body was destroying itself. It is a disease known as an autoimmune disease in which your own immune system turns against you. He was completely bedridden and unable to move even his fingers. He asked his doctor point-blank what his chances of recovery were. The doctor truthfully disclosed that the prognosis was very bad; the chances of recovery were less than 1 in 500, so bleak in fact that the news would send anyone into hopeless depression. But not Norman Cousins. He took a constructive view and asked himself what he could do to turn the odds in his favor?

His initial lines of thinking were: Why did he get this disease in the first place? What were the causes? He went over his life events preceding the illness, and he came to the conclusion that the stress of his travel abroad, intense work before and during the trip, being frustrated by bureaucracy and having to deal with incompetent people, exposure to fumes from diesel trucks driving nightly just outside his open bedroom window and accidentally being exposed to a stream of exhaust from the jet plane as he was embarking had probably lowered his resistance. It couldn't be the direct effect of toxic pollutants because his wife had been exposed to the same pollutants without any apparent harmful effects. He remembered reading in Hans Selye's classic book *The Stress of Life* (122) that emotional tension such as frustration or suppressed rage can cause adrenal exhaustion and lower the body's resistance to fight any kind of illness, including infection. He also remembered reading Walter B. Cannon's classic book *The Wisdom of the Body* (16a), in which he mentioned how the body, given half a chance, will work wonderfully well to maintain homeostasis or, in other words, to restore normal balance.

The next question was how to give that "half a chance" to the body, to boost his adrenal glands so they would fight off the disease and allow the body to heal itself. The enormous quantity of painkillers and anti-inflammatory drugs he was on (remember the doctors were fighting a life-and-death situation) was causing allergy, and he felt that perhaps, in his case, these tablets were doing more harm than good. He decided to put up with excruciating pain and reduce the tablets gradually with a view to stopping them. He also started on large doses of intravenous vitamin C, which he thought would help oxygenate his blood. Luckily his doctor was very sympathetic and cooperated fully. Cousins felt that positive emotions, like love, hope, faith, and laughter, were essential to enhance his body's fighting power. There were no problems with love, hope, and faith, he thought, but what about the laughter?

His friends sent him "Candid Camera" classics and old Marx Brothers films and they worked. He states "Ten minutes of belly laughter had an anaesthetic effect and would give me at least two hours of pain-free sleep. When the painkilling effect of the laughter wore off, we would switch on the motion-picture projector again, and, not infrequently, it would lead to another pain-free sleep interval." Sometimes the nurses would read him humor books. Within a week of this full-force laughter routine and vitamin C, he was completely off the drugs, including sleeping pills. On the eighth day he was able to move his thumb and he felt ecstatic. Gradually lumps on his neck and the backs of his hands began to shrink. It took many months for him to recover sufficiently to return to work and years to make a full recovery, but recover he did.

Did laughter contribute to his recovery? He certainly thought so. And the effect on his blood tests was the proof. After every laughter episode, his sedimentation rate would drop a few points. The sedimentation rate is the rate at which red cells settle down in a tube of blood. In a serious connective-tissue disease the sedimentation rate rises very high and a drop in the rate is a measure of progress in recovery. Some doctors thought that the drop was the effect of Cousins's belief in his own treatment, what scientists call a *placebo effect*. In other words, they questioned its scientific validity and felt that perhaps it was just a coincidence. If belief can be so powerful, then it behooves us to believe in ourselves: in the healing power of the brain and the life force, and in the benevolence of laughter.

ALTER YOUR PERSPECTIVE

Our personality, behavior patterns, and attitudes influence how we respond to stressful situations. We might not be able to remove those situations from our environment, but we can try to alter our negative attitudes and destructive behavior patterns.

The first important thing is to admit the existence of those attitudes and behavior patterns. Unfortunately, four out of five Type A people vehemently deny a Type A behavior pattern in themselves. The second important point is to believe that we can change our potentially destructive attitudes and behaviors. The third point is to work out positive steps and finally to put those steps into practice, accept some failings, but persevere and give ourselves a pat on the back for every success we have. The following are useful suggestions which, in fact, summarize most of the advice given in this book and are based on personal experiences as well as those of other authors listed in the references.

Fifty-Two Pearls of Wisdom

1. Learn to differentiate between minor irritations and major provocations and so not to respond to situations indiscriminately. All battles are not wars, and all wars are not nuclear wars (115).
2. Learn to become aware of your physical, behavioral, mental, and emotional tension levels and use stress management skills to control those tensions until your coping skills become second nature.

3. Use coping skills to prepare for stressful situations, as well as to meet those which come unexpectedly.

4. Feeling tired at the end of the day has nothing to do with what you have accomplished. It depends on how you have used your mind and body. If you are fatigued, you did not use them properly (19).

5. Just as you cannot learn to drive a car simply by reading a book or listening to a lecture, you cannot learn stress management until you regularly use stress management skills in real-life situations and are prepared to give yourself adequate opportunity to practice those skills.

6. Even though stress involves more than just bodily tension, physical relaxation is an important and effective stress management skill. Remember that tense muscles are working muscles. Ease up and save energy for more important things. Unclench your jaws, relax your shoulders, uncross your legs and relax your entire attitude while performing your daily tasks.

7. Even if you are feeling overwhelmed by multiple demands and insufficient time, the display of behavioral tension, such as in knee jiggling, finger tapping, using obscene language, and shouting at the secretary, can only make things worse.

8. Being irritable and impatient toward others leads them to mirror the response and thus creates a negative spiral of escalating tension. The very act of banging on the table or shouting at a colleague increases the stress we are already experiencing.

9. Be yourself and act like yourself. The biggest mistake behind so much misery is our longing to be someone other than ourselves. Many a successful person has learned this lesson early in his career.

10. It is not advisable to rant and rave when you are upset. The damage caused by such a display will require too much energy and time to repair (115).

11. It is inappropriate either to bottle up emotion or to lose emotional control. What you should do is use an effective communication skill.

12. By speaking in a calm, modulated voice, adopting a physically relaxed posture, and listening attentively to people, you can improve your interactions with others as well as increase your sense of well-being.

13. All of us experience frustrations, conflict, disappointment, and defeat at some time or other in our personal or professional lives. However, it is up to you how you interpret and react to these feelings.

14. Learn to count your blessings, not your misfortunes. Do you have a shelter to live under? Sufficient food and clothes? Eyes and ears with which to see and hear? Would you sell your eyes for a million dollars? A leg for ten thousand dollars? You are not poor then. Indeed, you have priceless assets (19).

15. Our reactions depend on our attitudes and beliefs. Having a perfectionist attitude ("I must always be perfect in everything I do") is unrealistic and leads to unnecessary stress.

16. Do not couch thoughts in a negative blanket. Self-talk like "It shouldn't have happened," "I can't understand it," and "It's horrible" again leads to unnecessary stress (31).

17. Do not put yourself down with statements like "I am so stupid, I can't do anything right," which put your self-worth into question. We all can make a mistake sometimes. One mistake doesn't make you a failure.

18. Many stressful situations are regular occurrences in life, like the line in a supermarket, hostile cracks by a colleague at a regular meeting, the time pressure of meeting frequent deadlines, or commuting to work. Anticipating them and either avoiding them or taking effective preventive action can significantly reduce stress levels.

19. Each one of us has his own idiosyncratic stress signals telling him he is out of control. They should be used as a reminder to take one deep breath and let go of physical tension.

20. By using behavior which is incompatible with stress signs, you can defuse the disturbance created by stress (115). Thus, speaking slowly whenever you find yourself shouting or breathing deeply whenever you are tense will defuse the situation.

21. Before you dominate a conversation, ask yourself, "Do I really have something to say? Does anyone wish to hear it and is this the right time to say it?" (38)

22. Remind yourself that few ventures fail because we are slow. Good judgment and correct decisions require deliberation, not haste (38).

23. Expecting yourself to have completed all your projects at a given time is unrealistic and sure to lead to stress.

24. Remind yourself that giving and receiving love are not a sign of weakness but the source of spiritual strength that we have all been seeking unconsciously since childhood.

25. Find ways to give and receive love. Express your appreciation with flowers. Thank-you letters or a small unexpected gift encourage others to return the kindness.

26. Regularly expressing your love and affection to your spouse and children is likely to make them feel warmer toward you.

27. Be ready to help your friends in any way and every way you can, but refrain from giving unsought advice.

28. When we feel good about ourselves, the irritations of life do not bother us so much. For example, it is almost impossible to pick a quarrel with your spouse if you have just received a raise in salary or a pro-

motion. Try to keep your self-image high through positive self-dialogue.

29. In order to increase your coping resilience, you should strive for a positive self-image. Statements like "I did a pretty good job considering the difficulties" tend to boost the morale.

30. Physical relaxation, adequate sleep, prudent diet, and regular exercise can increase coping resilience. You should plan for regular pleasurable activities just as you plan and execute work obligations. A slogan popularized by Ethel Roskies is "A pleasure a day keeps the stress away" (115).

31. Little courteous phrases like "I am so sorry to trouble you," "Would you be so kind . . . ," "Would you mind . . . ," "Thank you," and "Won't you please . . . ," show your respect for others. They are also tremendously potent in getting people to cooperate (19).

32. A sure way to reach people's hearts is to convey in some subtle way that you appreciate their talents or recognize their importance. If you succeed in making people feel important, they will go out of their way to help you.

33. It is easy to become addicted to stress hormones like epinephrine and norepinephrine. Many physicians feel that coronary patients seem to be "hooked on adrenaline" prior to their heart attacks.

34. Hostile Type A individuals, say Meyer Friedman and Diane Ulmer (38), not only expect their environment to present them with absolute truths and certitudes but also strive to erase doubts and uncertainty from their own thoughts and actions. Such attitudes irritate and antagonize friends and family.

35. Don't fall into the trap of trying to be perfect. As Robert Eliot and Dennis Breo, the authors of *Is It Worth Dying For?* said, "Perfectionism is self-destruc-

tive because you have made the game impossible to win" (31).

36. Be guided by your own feelings and not by what others might say. Your self-image and feeling of personal worth come from within.

37. If you treat work as your be-all and end-all, your life is not very well balanced. A career can certainly be a source of fulfillment, but it can also become an escape from other responsibilities.

38. To balance life you need to build some fun and play into your daily schedule. Take a long weekend break or a halfday off to play golf, or spend an evening out at the theater.

39. Take thirty-second breaks several times a day. For example, when you are driving, take one deep breath and relax at every red traffic light, or when a telephone rings, relax with a deep breath, compose yourself, and only then pick it up.

40. Drive slowly in the right-hand lane. If you find this difficult, listen to soothing music while driving to reduce your urge to drive faster and faster.

41. Interrupt long sessions of work with short breaks every hour or two. Stretch out, stroke a pet, sip mineral water or tea, or talk to a colleague.

42. Learn to accept things which can't be changed. There is no point in getting upset over and over again about circumstances or other people's behavior which are beyond your control.

43. Review the causes of your feelings of time urgency and make plans for effective management. If you feel that you don't have time to practice your stress management strategies, you'll certainly have trouble getting things done, because it will be harder for you to define priorities and you will find yourself going around in circles.

44. Stop for a minute or two several times a day. Look at yourself, your behavior, and your relationships, and ask yourself how you can take better care of yourself and listen to your inner wisdom. With this "stop, look, and listen" technique you will almost always find an answer within yourself (62).

45. Taking good care of yourself will make you take better care of your business and family.

46. Develop a sense of humor and learn to laugh at follies and imperfections. Laughing makes you feel healthy, happy, and humane. Listening to a comedy tape can wipe out blues.

47. You can be your best friend or worst enemy. What will it be? Instead of being miserable for what you don't have, be thankful for what you do have. Pain comes from not appreciating what you do have and thinking about what you should have.

48. If you want people to give you loyalty and cooperation, make them feel important. The deepest principle in human nature is the craving to be appreciated.

49. Ask yourself if what you are chasing is something you really want. Spending your time and energy chasing after things you don't really need in the first place is likely to disappoint you and drain you of vitality.

50. Learning new habits takes time. We all need to practice and persevere. At times we will revert back to our old ways, but we should not lose heart. Learn and relearn as often as is necessary. There is a saying, "God helps them who help themselves."

51. When we grow apart in marriage or other relationships there is a tendency to believe that we could be happy if only the other were more considerate. The secret lies in loving yourself. When you are happy within yourself, you automatically give the other the love, tenderness, respect, and attention he or she deserves.

52. Even more important than being loved is being lov-
    ing, says Spencer Johnson, the author of *One Minute
    for Myself* (62).

14

Nutrition and a Healthy Lifestyle

Certain habits increase susceptibility to stress. They generally include cigarette smoking; eating too much or eating the wrong food; excessive drinking of coffee, tea, or alcohol; and dependence on tranquilizers, sleeping pills, and other medications. Proper nutrition and adopting healthy habits can increase resistance to stress as well as directly reduce the risk of illness.

NUTRITION

What we eat matters considerably in maintaining health and preventing disease. When our nutrition is good, our organs, muscles, and tissues are healthy. Our energy level is high, our bodies are strong and resistant to adverse effects of the environment, and our minds are clear. When nutrition is defective, we can be susceptible to every kind of illness. Many diseases of modern society, including obesity, arthritis, coronary heart disease, cancer of the bowel, diverticulosis, constipation, diabetes, migraine, and even unlikely things like varicose veins have their roots in the type of foods we eat and the way they are processed. This knowledge has brought a new surge of interest in nutrition. The idea that we need so many grams of protein, carbohydrate, and fats and so many milligrams of each of the vitamins and minerals is giving way to the feeling that perhaps we do not know everything there is to know about nutrition and that we need to eat varied and wholesome foods with a minimum of processing and preservatives to ensure that we get everything we need, known and unknown, without the possible harmful effects of additives.

Modern progress in preserving, canning, processing, and producing foods has certainly added an enormous variety of convenience foods to our tables, but certain methods have proved harmful to health, and the safety of others has yet to be proven. Chemical sprays and fertilizers are used with alarming casualness in farming. Gases are used to ripen and preserve fruit and vegetables. We each consume, it is suggested, two to five pounds of additives a year! Of course there have been enormous advantages, too. In many industrialized countries, where most people live far away from agricultural areas, preserving and freezing ensures that most of us get fresh, uncontaminated foods. We should not get fanatical but should have a sense of proportion, and we should get into the habit of reading labels and whenever possible using fresh foods. Did you know that fruit and vegetables stored at room temperature may lose up to 70 percent of their vitamins A, C, and D in about three days? Our biggest problem, however, is that we eat too much animal fat—what the nutritionists call *saturated fat*—and not enough foods containing omega-3 fatty acids, found in fish as well as fresh fruit and vegetables, and we consume an inadequate quantity of fiber.

Saturated Fat and Cholesterol

The consumption of fat in Western countries is very high. For example, in North America, the average consumption is

100 grams (4 oz.) a day. A healthy adult needs no more than 75 grams (3 oz.) per day. Therefore, consumption should be cut by at least a quarter. However, the problem with fat is not that simple, because the type of fat in the diet is also important. There are three main categories of fat found in the diet: saturated, monounsaturated, and polyunsaturated.

Saturated fat tends to encourage the liver to produce cholesterol and to make the blood more prone to clot. Polyunsaturated fat, on the other hand, tends to lower the level of total cholesterol in the blood and may even reduce the stickiness of the blood particles known as *platelets*. Polyunsaturated fat, therefore, plays a protective role in helping to keep the walls of the arteries clear. Monounsaturated fat does not increase cholesterol, but neither does it reduce it. More recent evidence, however, suggests that monounsaturated fat, like olive oil and peanut oil, is in fact beneficial.

Not only is our consumption of fat very high and, therefore, an important contributory factor to obesity, but more than half of all fat consumed is saturated. Cutting down on fat generally can stop, and may actually reverse, existing atherosclerosis (hardening of the arteries). It is particularly important to reduce the amount of saturated fat in your diet and to make sure that the fat you do eat is, as far as possible, polyunsaturated. Recent research work by Ornish and his colleagues (95a) has shown significant unblocking of the coronary arteries of those with documented coronary artery disease when they reduce their fat intake to less than 1 oz. per day and regularly practice stress management techniques.

Which Food Contains Saturated Fat? No one food contains only a single type of fat; it is the relative proportion of the different types of fat within a food that makes the food healthy or unhealthy. In general, saturated fat tends to be solid at room temperature and comes from animal sources, whereas polyunsaturated fat is soft, or in the form of oil, and comes from vegetables and fish.

Saturated fat is found in beef, lamb, pork, and in processed meat products such as bacon, sausages, and frankfurters. Hamburger bought from a supermarket usually has a rather high fat content. You can avoid this source of fat by buying lean meat and chopping it yourself.

Poultry, or white meat, contains less fat than red meat, especially when the skin is removed. Game, such as rabbit, venison, pigeon, and pheasant, is the leanest meat of all and contains much more polyunsaturated fat and less saturated fat than other meat. Duck and goose are fatty meats, but the fat is rather less saturated than the fat in red meat.

Milk and most dairy products, such as butter, full-fat cheese, and cream, are high in saturated fat.

High levels of cholesterol are found in eggs, liver, kidney, heart, brain, and shrimp and other shellfish.

Oils which are low in saturates and high in polyunsaturates include (in descending order of polyunsaturated fat content) safflower, soybean, sunflower, corn, cottonseed, and sesame. Olive oil and peanut oil contain monounsaturated fat.

But beware: just because a food label tells you that a food contains vegetable oil it does not necessarily mean that it is free from saturated fat. Coconut oil, cocoa butter, and palm oil (used in commercially prepared biscuits, pie fillings, and nondairy milk and cream substitutes) are all saturated fats. Avoid blended oils because they can be high in saturates.

Even a naturally healthy, polyunsaturated oil can be turned into a harmful, saturated fat if artificially hardened, a process known as hydrogenation. All margarine, for example, contains some hydrogenated fat or it would spill out of the tub. It is a question of degree: the harder the margarine, the more saturated and less healthy it is. Margarine which is labeled "high in polyunsaturates" must contain at least 40 percent of its total fat content as polyunsaturates. Always buy "cold-pressed" oil because it is extracted from the fresh, raw seed; the heat treatment used in some forms of processing can convert some of the polyunsaturated fat into saturated fat.

The Advantages of Fish. White fish contains hardly any fat at all and is a high-protein, low-fat alternative to meat. Fatty fish, such as mackerel, herring, sardines, tuna, salmon, and trout, are excellent sources of polyunsaturated oil. This oil contains omega-3 fatty acid, which is believed to have a particularly protective effect on the circulation by making the blood platelets less sticky and consequently less liable to clot. One of the reasons why Eskimos have a low incidence of heart disease is thought to be the large amount of fish they eat. The Japanese, too, eat more fish than we do in the West, and they, too, are known to have a very low rate of coronary heart disease.

It is a good idea, therefore, to eat fish at least two or three times every week, including fatty fish at least once, and if you eat canned fish, such as sardines or tuna, choose ones in a named, healthy oil, such as soybean or olive.

Tips for Cutting Down on Saturated Fats

- Eat poultry and game in preference to red meat and meat products. Remove the skin from chicken and other poultry.
- Eat more fish.
- If you do eat red meat, trim away any fat before cooking.
- Grill or bake rather than fry. Cook meat on a rack so that the fat can drain.
- If you do fry, use polyunsaturated oil, rather than butter or lard, and a nonstick pan so that you use only a very small amount of oil to prevent sticking.
- Bought ground meat often contains a lot of fat, so it's best to buy lean stewing beef. Cut off all visible fat and grind the meat yourself. Fry the ground meat or ham-

burger without adding any fat and then drain off all the fat before you add flavorings.

- Use polyunsaturated margarine instead of butter and spread it sparingly.
- Avoid hard cheese, such as cheddar and Stilton, and cream cheese, and buy lower fat cheeses, such as Edam, Camembert, or other low-fat hard cheese or, even better, cottage or curd cheese as an alternative.
- Change from full-fat milk to semiskimmed or, best of all, skimmed.
- Use plain low-fat yogurt instead of cream, mayonnaise, or sour cream.
- Boil or poach eggs (and no more than three a week) rather than scrambling or frying them with butter.
- Eat more vegetarian meals or stretch meat by mixing it with legumes and vegetables.
- Eat baked or boiled potatoes in preference to french fries.
- Avoid manufactured food, such as cookies, cake, pastry, sauces, and chips, which are rich in "hidden" fat, usually saturated. If you must eat cake, make your own using a healthy, polyunsaturated fat.

Vegetarianism

This is not simply a matter of cutting meat from the diet. Vegetarianism involves adding nutritious alternatives like seeds, grains, nuts, legumes, cereals, and sprouts. A well-balanced diet including the above, as well as plenty of fresh fruit and vegetables, is as nutritious as a well-planned nonvegetarian diet containing meat. In addition to supplying adequate proteins, carbohydrates, fats, vitamins, and minerals, a well-balanced vegetarian diet also supplies a good measure of fiber, now considered beneficial to health.

Fiber

Fiber is the name given to a range of complex carbohydrates found in the cell walls of plants. Also known as *roughage*, it provides bulk and prevents constipation and other intestinal disorders like irritable bowel and diverticulosis. Fiber passes through the bowel without being absorbed and, as it hastens the passage of food through the bowel, it reduces the absorption of harmful cholesterol and sugar and even of carcinogenic substances. By controlling sugar and cholesterol levels, fiber benefits us by preventing diabetes and atherosclerosis. Foods which are high in fiber include bananas, brown rice, potatoes in their skins, dried fruits, leafy vegetables, legumes, oatmeal, sweet corn, whole-grain bread, whole wheat pasta, and rhubarb. Bran is mostly fiber.

Sugar

Despite widespread knowledge that sugar rots teeth and contributes to obesity, sugar consumption remains high in the Western world. Less than half the sugar consumed is bought as bags of sugar; the rest comes in candy, cake, carbonated drinks, and processed foods.

Sugar is thought by some researchers to contribute to the risk of coronary heart disease, though no one knows for certain why this should be so. The evidence is partly confounded by the fact that those who consume sugar also eat a lot of fat, for instance, in cakes, which causes an increase in the level of blood cholesterol. Some recent research has also suggested that excess sugar is turned in the liver into fat, most of which is saturated.

One point on which researchers are certain is that most of us need to reduce the amount of sugar we eat. This includes not only packaged sugar, whether white, brown, or raw unrefined cane or beet sugar, but also sugar in processed foods, where it might be listed as sugar, sucrose, syrup, dextrose, molasses, or caramel. If you must eat sweeteners, use honey or fruit juice concentrates, which contain the natural sugars fructose and glucose, as well as minerals and vitamins.

Tips for Cutting Down on Sugar

- Drink unsweetened fruit juices, diluted with mineral water if necessary.
- Do not eat candy and other sweets.
- Eat fruit at the end of a meal rather than a sticky dessert, and munch a piece of fruit as a snack rather than candy or chocolate.
- Halve the amount of sugar in recipes.
- Read the list of ingredients on all processed foods, and do not buy them if they contain sugar.

Salt

An adult needs to eat only 1 gram of salt a day but many of us consume far more. For example, in North America, we eat about 10 grams (1/3 oz.) of salt, or sodium chloride, a day. All fruit, vegetables, milk, meat, and cereal contain small amounts of sodium. We get enough from these sources, and the addition of extra salt is unnecessary unless we are involved in strenuous or athletic activity which causes us to perspire freely.

A high consumption of salt is thought by many doctors to be a risk factor in high blood pressure which is, in turn, a risk factor in coronary heart disease and strokes. Most healthy people can get rid of excess sodium through the kidneys and it does not cause them any harm. However, some people are sensitive to sodium, and it is in these people that excessive sodium may cause high blood pressure.

The Problem of Hidden Salt. About three-quarters of the salt we eat is added to processed food, which also contains sodium in many other guises: monosodium glutamate (flavor enhancer); sodium bicarbonate (baking soda); sodium cyclamate and sodium saccharin (artificial sweeteners); and sodium nitrate, sodium sulfite, and sodium benzoate (preservatives). Look out for anything with the word *sodium* or its chemical symbol *Na* in the list of ingredients. Some over-the-counter medicine also contains sodium without its being on the label. Salt added at home accounts for the rest of our salt intake and this is something we can easily control ourselves.

Tips for Cutting Down on Salt

- Start by adding salt either during cooking or at the table, never both. Then, as your taste buds adapt, gradually cut down the amount further.
- Use salt substitutes or low-sodium salt or alternative flavoring such as lemon juice, spices, or herbs.
- Avoid highly salted food such as salami, bacon, ham, sausages, frankfurters, potato chips, bouillon cubes, processed cheese, salted nuts, pickles, olives, ketchup, soy sauce, and smoked fish.
- Keep an eye on your children's eating habits, as a taste for oversalted food is acquired early in life. Never give salt to babies or toddlers, whose kidneys are too immature to deal with it.
- Artificially softened water contains more sodium than hard water, so if you use a domestic water softener, make sure you have a drinking tap for water without softener.
- Read all food and over-the-counter medicine labels carefully for salt content.

MAINTAINING IDEAL BODY WEIGHT

Obesity

Stress can make us fat as people often eat for comfort, and obesity can increase our stress because slimness is equated with beauty while obesity is equated with gluttony, sloth, and ugliness. The guilt associated with such feelings can turn us to food for comfort and a vicious circle is perpetuated. Reasons for overeating include the following:

- To diminish anxiety, insecurity, tension, worry, or indecision; to achieve pleasure, gratification, or success
- To express hostility, conscious or unconscious, denied or repressed
- To reward oneself
- To diminish guilt, including guilt due to overeating

Unfortunately the explanations offered are often contradictory. Some people eat because their parents didn't love them enough; others eat because their parents loved them too much. People eat when they are angry and they eat when they are bored. Some eat to celebrate joy. Whatever the cause, obesity certainly leads to stress because of the social stigma attached to it.

In addition to its psychological disadvantage, being overweight is associated with poor health. If you weigh a fifth or more in excess of your ideal weight you are more likely to suffer from fatigue, accidents, acid indigestion, hernia, flat feet, arthritis, varicose veins, and, even more serious, high blood pressure, diabetes, or heart attack. The tendency to gain excess weight may be inherited, but this fact does not help you in controlling your weight. To lose weight, you have either to eat fewer calories than you burn or to increase your energy output by exercise in relation to your energy intake. In practice, the most effective way of losing weight is by both eating fewer calories and increasing the amount of exercise you take.

Ideal Body Weight Chart. Measure your height without shoes, and weigh yourself without clothes. If you weigh more than the maximum weight for your height and sex, you may be seriously overweight.

Height	Acceptable weight	
	Men	Women
1.57m (5ft 2ins)	–	46-59kg (102-131lb)
1.60m (5ft 3ins)	–	48-61kg (105-134lb)
1.63m (5ft 4ins)	54-67kg (118-148lb)	49-63kg (108-138lb)
1.65m (5ft 5ins)	65-69kg (121-152lb)	50-64kg (111-142lb)
1.68m (5ft 6ins)	56-71kg (124-156lb)	52-66kg (114-146lb)
1.70m (5ft 7ins)	58-73kg (128-161lb)	54-68kg (118-150lb)
1.73m (5ft 8ins)	60-75kg (132-166lb)	55-70kg (122-154lb)
1.75m (5ft 9ins)	62-77kg (136-170lb)	57-72kg (126-158lb)
1.78m (5ft 10ins)	64-79kg (140-173lb)	59-74kg (130-163lb)
1.80m (5ft 11ins)	65-81kg (144-179lb)	61-76kg (134-168lb)
1.83m (6ft)	67-83kg (148-184lb)	63-78kg (138-173lb)
1.85m (6ft 1in)	69-86kg (152-189lb)	–
1.88m (6ft 2ins)	71-88kg (156-194lb)	–
1.90m (6ft 3ins)	73-90kg (160-199lb)	

Tips for Losing Weight

One of the benefits of eating the low-fat, low-sugar, high-fiber diet already mentioned, in addition to limiting your alcohol intake and increasing your physical activity, is that it helps you to keep slim and avoid obesity. Not everyone who eats a lot puts on weight. Unfortunately, however, some people have a slow metabolism, which tends to run in families, and will put on weight on a diet which other people can enjoy without putting on an ounce. However, this understanding does not help you much if you tend to put on weight easily because your problem is still that you are eating more than you are burning up or that you are eating more than you need for the amount of activity you pursue. If you need to lose weight, reduce drastically your intake of the following:

- Butter, margarine, cooking fats, oils, and fried food
- Cheese and cream
- Fatty meat
- Pastry, cookies, cake, nuts, and chips
- Rich sauces and soups
- Sugary foods, including jam, honey, candy, and chocolate
- Alcohol

Several small meals are better than one or two heavy meals, and you should stop eating when you feel satisfied. Don't be tempted to clean up your plate and don't allow yourself to be very hungry since you will be tempted to snack on readily available foods like cookies and cake. You may find it helpful to arm yourself with a book on weight loss or a calorie guide, to join a weight-loss club, or to ask your doctor for advice, but don't ask him to prescribe diet pills as they are harmful and not effective in the long run.

How to Stick to a Weight-Loss Diet

Most diet pamphlets tell you what to eat and what not to eat. Unfortunately they do not tell you how to resist temptation, bearing in mind that eating is a pleasurable occupation which fulfills not only nutritional requirements but also social and psychological needs (34).

Parties and Eating Out. When eating out choose sensible items. A melon or fruit cocktail could be eaten as a starter instead of a paté, resist eating a roll and butter while waiting for the first course to be served, choose fish or chicken for the main course but not in rich sauces, and have salad or boiled vegetables instead of French fries. Tell the waiter you do not want butter on your vegetables, as vegetables are often served dripping with butter, and avoid oily or creamy salad dressing. Fruit salad or strawberries are a good choice for dessert but do avoid cream. If you must eat something sweeter, crème caramel or a small portion of ice cream might be your next alternative.

At a party, drink mineral water or fruit juice instead of alcohol or have one drink and sip slowly to make it last the whole evening. Allow yourself a limited number of canapes. Avoid piling food on your plate at a buffet party. To avoid this, first walk from one end to the other end of the table to see what is there, and then choose only items you would really enjoy. There is no need to be a martyr and deny yourself everything because you will only go home feeling completely deprived and upset and probably console yourself with a box of chocolates!

Psychological Need for Food. People sometimes eat to satisfy a psychological need. If you eat when your mind is occupied, such as while reading or watching television, the food will not satisfy your psychological need and you will be tempted to eat more. To gain the full benefit of eating put your book down or turn off the television and concentrate on your food, relishing each mouthful.

Food Craving. If you get a craving for a particular high-calorie food which you know you shouldn't eat, don't give in immediately. Once the critical period passes, you often lose the craving. However, if the craving persists at the end of the day or if it is still there the next morning, it is better to satisfy it with a small portion of the food in question than to let it intensify to the extent where you are in danger of losing all control. One woman in three has cravings for sweet food three or four days before her period. If you have this problem, either satisfy yourself with low-calorie foods or substitute craved-for foods with normal meals.

Diversionary Tactics. You may find yourself turning to food for comfort whenever you feel frustrated or angry. Persuade yourself to wait for fifteen minutes. Once your emotions are in control you may not feel the need to eat. If you tend to eat when feeling sorry for yourself or when bored, busy yourself with some task that you have been putting off for a long time. You will be surprised how a sense of accomplishment can lift your mood and alleviate your desire for food. Do shopping after a meal so that you won't be tempted to buy those ready-to-eat cream cakes or other high-calorie foods or to eat on your way home. Make a shopping list and restrict yourself to only those items which are on the list.

Eating without Knowing. The subconscious can sometimes play amazing tricks on your mind. You may, for example, eat something you are not supposed to on your diet, then forget all about it. One way of combating this is to write down everything you eat and drink throughout the day. The most important thing to remember is not to set yourself unrealistic, overoptimistic goals. This is the downfall of many a slimmer. There are bound to be occasions when it is simply not possible to observe a diet rigorously. Accept that the occasional slip-up is a necessary part of learning a new eating pattern.

Self-Hypnosis. Almost any habit can be controlled if you have sufficient motivation. Self-hypnosis is particularly good for helping you to stick to a diet. Try the following sequence two or three times a day, preferably before each meal (123):

- Sit in a comfortable chair, close your eyes, and deeply relax.
- Repeat one or more of the following phrases to yourself ten to twenty times: "I can see and feel myself as happy and healthy," "I can see my body clearly," or "I undress and look at my body in a full-length mirror."

- Next repeat five to ten times as many of the following phrases as you can remember: "Now I can see and feel my body at my ideal weight," "My appetite is pleasantly satisfied," "I become increasingly comfortable as I attain my desired weight," "I become healthier and healthier as I attain my desired weight," "I feel happy and proud of myself as I attain my desired weight," "I am satisfied with small portions of food," and "I can see and feel my body at my ideal weight and I will carry this image and feeling with me as I return to my normal awareness."

- As you prepare to return to your normal awareness, take a deep breath, open your eyes, stretch comfortably, and continue to feel gloriously happy, completely satisfied, and full of energy.

Anorexia and Bulimia

Many people, especially women, because it is socially desirable, keep themselves thin but pay a high emotional price for being fashionably gaunt. They make a fetish of being thin and follow a weight-reducing diet with little awareness of or regard to their health, because by not permitting themselves to eat properly they drive themselves into continuous tension and strain, irritability, and poor physical health. Some become so preoccupied with this goal that they are unable to follow educational or professional careers. Chronic dieting makes us hungry because the brain doesn't recognize that we are dieting voluntarily. So, whether crash dieting or constantly attempting to hold eating in check, we are bound to feel hungry. When restraint is no longer possible, as will be the case from time to time, dieters go on a binge and eat until they can eat no more. Following the binge, they feel so guilty that they either take regular doses of purgative medicine or physically make themselves sick. The constant conflict between the physical desire to eat because of hunger and the mind's obsession with remaining thin leads to overeating and then vomiting—the condition known as *bulimia*. Sometimes the obsession distorts the image of the body, and these thin people, still thinking they are too fat, continue to restrict their food intake, deny that they are hungry and in the process become emaciated—the condition popularly known as *anorexia*.

SMOKING

There is only one sensible thing to do about smoking—QUIT. Tobacco smoke is a complex mixture of some 4,000 chemicals, of which the most significant are nicotine and carbon monoxide. Two to three drops of pure nicotine alcohol on the tongue will kill an adult in minutes. A typical cigarette contains 15 to 20 milligrams of nicotine, although the actual amount reaching the blood varies, depending on the type of filter, the depth and frequency of inhalation, and the length of the butt.

Long-Term Effects of Smoking

Long-term smoking increases the danger of:

- Heart attack
- Stroke
- Lung cancer
- Chronic bronchitis
- Exacerbation of asthma
- Stomach ulcer
- Premature birth
- Miscarriage or stillbirth
- Mental or physical developmental defects of unborn babies
- Vitamin C depletion

- Impaired healing of skin wounds or ulcers
- Release of excessive stress hormone
- Bad breath
- Nicotine stains on fingers
- Poor digestion
- Poor appetite

Rationalization

People continue to smoke, despite health warnings on each package of cigarettes, because of the particular kind of logic which they use to justify their habit. Examples of rationalization are:

- Uncle John smoked a pack a day and lived to be a hundred.
- I don't have the willpower.
- If I stop smoking, I will put on weight.
- Smoking helps me to relax.
- Smoking helps me to concentrate.
- I have smoked for many years. Isn't it too late to stop?
- I don't smoke as much as I used to.
- I don't really inhale, so it can't be very bad.
- I have tried hundreds of times before but I can't stick to it.
- I become irritable when I stop, so my spouse won't like it.
- At least I am not harming others.
- If I am going to die, I could be run over by a bus.

Useful Tips for Giving Up

Nobody says it is easy to give up, but hundreds of people have done it, so you can, too. You may find the following hints useful:

- Throw away cigarettes and all smoking paraphernalia.
- Don't sit around after a meal.
- Take a few deep breaths when you have an urge to smoke.
- Give up with a partner or a friend and then support each other.
- Let other people know that you have given up smoking.
- Write down all the positive things about nonsmoking.
- Write down all the reasons for giving up smoking.
- Suck a mint, chew gum, or nibble a carrot when you have an urge to smoke.
- Try chewing nicotine chewing gum every time you have the urge.
- Think of the amount of money you will save over a year.

Giving Up in Stages

Start with giving up one of the cigarettes from the following list and then give up others gradually:

- Do not smoke in bed.
- Do not smoke first thing in the morning.
- Do not smoke before breakfast.
- Do not smoke while traveling.
- Do not smoke before a meal.
- Do not smoke during a meal.
- Do not smoke a whole cigarette.
- Do not smoke more than one cigarette an hour.
- Do not smoke before going to bed.

Relaxed Persuasion

Sit quietly for five minutes and relax all your muscles. Close your eyes and mentally repeat one or more of the following phrases fifteen to twenty times:

- Smoking doesn't matter. I can breathe better in fresh air.
- I am becoming freer and freer from nicotine and feeling happier and happier.
- I am in perfect control of my health and proud of my accomplishment.
- I am calm and relaxed and free from cigarettes.

ALCOHOL

Alcoholic drinks have been enjoyed since the beginning of recorded history. So what's wrong with them? The answer is simply that there is nothing wrong with drinking moderate amounts. In many Western nations, almost two-thirds of adults drink. Only 10 percent of them develop a problem. There is no need for moderate drinkers to jump on the dry wagon. In California, Hales and Hales reported (47) that moderate drinkers lived seven to eleven years longer than those who didn't drink at all. In a study of 17,249 Canadians, those who drank a pint of beer a day had 28 percent fewer illnesses than the average (47). Moderate drinkers have fewer heart attacks than heavy drinkers or those who abstain, although there is no evidence that taking up moderate drinking for the first time will necessarily reduce your risk. Recently doubt has been raised on this issue as some believe that in research studies a number of abstainers are actually ex-drinkers who probably have given up drinking for health reasons; thus they help inflate the risk of true teetotalers. If modest drinking is beneficial, as is claimed, how does this benefit from moderate drinking accrue? Researchers think that a moderate amount of alcohol boosts our high-density lipoprotein (HDL), the good part of cholesterol. Recently it has been reported that alcohol increases our blood level of Apo-A lipoprotein, which clears our blood of cholesterol. Moderate drinking does not reduce our brainpower provided we stick to our limit, although it is best not to drink at a time when the mind needs to be crystal clear.

What Is Moderate or Heavy Drinking?

Moderate drinking	Men: Up to twenty-one drinks per week
	Women: Up to fifteen drinks per week
Heavy drinking	Men: More than fifty-one drinks per week
	Women: More than thirty-six drinks per week

Because you are allowed fifteen or twenty-one drinks a week, it doesn't mean that you can save up all your allowance and have a binge on Sunday. You must spread your drinking throughout the week. About two drinks a day seems to be optimum. Those who drink between three and five drinks a day have a 50 percent higher mortality rate than those who drink two drinks or less per day. Those who drink five or more drinks a day have five times the risk of dying prematurely of teetotalers.

What Is a Standard Drink?

- Half-pint of beer or lager
- Third-pint of hard cider
- 1 oz. spirit (bourbon, Scotch, gin, brandy, vodka, rum)
- 4 oz. table wine
- 2.5 oz. sherry or port

Not all drinks have the same potency and it is important to know the type you drink in order to assess the real quantity you consume.

In addition to knowing the potency and the quantity of your drink, there are other factors you need to know. Women can hold less drink than men because of their lesser amount of body water. A hefty, muscular man can tolerate a larger amount than a thin man. Eating food, particularly high-protein foods, will slow down alcohol absorption from the stomach. If you drink a straight shot, it will reach your bloodstream quicker than if you mix your drink with water or fruit juice. Older people have less body water than young people and their blood level of alcohol will be higher after a similar drink.

HOW DIFFERENT DRINKS COMPARE

	Type of drink	Quantity	Standard drink equivalent
Beers and lagers	Ordinary strength beer or lager	½ pint	1
		1 pint	2
		1 12-oz. can	1½
	Strong ale or lager	½ pint	2
		1 pint	4
		1 12-oz. can	3
	Extra-strength beer or lager	½ pint	2½
		1 pint	6
		1 12-oz. can	4
Ciders	Ordinary strength	½ pint	1½
		1 pint	3
	Strong cider	½ pint	2
		1 pint	4
Spirits	Scotch, gin, bourbon, brandy, rum, vodka	1-oz. measure	1-1½
		1 bottle	30
Wines	Table wine	1 glass (4 oz.)	1
		1 bottle (700 cl)	7
		1 liter	10
	Sherry, port, vermouth	1 measure	1
		1 bottle	10

What Can Heavy Drinking Lead To?

- Alcohol dependency
- Vitamin B deficiency
- Rise in blood pressure
- Obesity
- Increased tendency to stroke
- Cirrhosis of the liver
- Increased risk of developing cancers of the throat, mouth, stomach, and lungs
- Road traffic accidents
- Pneumonia
- Suicide
- May cause death if combined with tranquilizers, sleeping pills, antihistamines (cold and allergy remedies), marijuana, or barbiturates
- Congenital defects or brain damage in unborn babies

How to Reduce Your Drinking Habits

- Avoid the situations in which you are most likely to drink. For example, leave work early or late to avoid your usual time for a drink.
- Avoid the company of the person with whom you usually have heavy drinking sessions.
- Sip your drink slowly to make it last longer.
- Avoid the habit of buying rounds.
- Limit yourself to smaller measures of drink.
- Arrive late at cocktail parties and leave early.
- Tell your drinking friends you are saving money, trying to lose weight, driving, or acting on doctor's orders.

Relaxed Persuasion

Try the following exercise two to three times a day or whenever you feel like having a drink (123).

Sit quietly and relax your muscles. When you are feeling completely relaxed repeat one or more of the following phrases mentally fifteen to twenty times:

- "I am becoming freer and freer from alcohol and feeling happier and happier every day."
- "As each day goes by, I am able to abstain from alcohol for longer and longer periods."
- "I am in perfect control of my drinking and I am proud of this."
- "I am calm and relaxed and free from alcohol."

As you prepare to return to your normal awareness, imagine feeling full of health and happiness. Take a deep breath, stretch your body, and feel refreshed, full of energy, and completely at peace with yourself.

Getting Outside Help

Cutting down gradually is much easier if you have the support of your family and friends. If you live on your own, or if you have had trouble cutting down in the past, you may benefit from outside help. Talk to your doctor, who, depending upon the extent of your problem, may decide to refer you to one of the many centers that help people get off and stay off alcohol. In some cases a course of hypnosis or acupuncture might help. Ask your doctor if he can refer you to one. If you are a heavy drinker and have tried to give up unsuccessfully in the past or you need to stop alcohol for some other medical condition, your doctor may arrange for you to be admitted to hospital for "drying out." If this happens, you will probably be treated as follows.

During the first day you will be given six drinks, a large dose of tranquilizer, and an anticonvulsant drug to keep you from having fits. The number of drinks you are allowed will be reduced by one every day, and the amount of tranquilizer and anticonvulsant drug will also be reduced proportionately.

Your stay in the hospital will range from ten days to four weeks, and before you are discharged from the hospital you will be put in touch with your local branch of Alcoholics Anonymous or a similar organization. These organizations have a 24-hour telephone number which you can use any time you need help or support. They also arrange regular meetings where you can discuss your problem with professional counselors or other people who have successfully stopped drinking, and of course you will meet other people who are in the same boat as you, so you won't feel that you are the only unfortunate person.

CAFFEINE

Caffeine is the drug that gives coffee its stimulating property. What is not widely known, however, is that caffeine is also found to some extent in tea, colas, and chocolate. People are often surprised when reducing the amount of coffee they drink relieves their heart palpitations and improves the depth of their sleep. Caffeine increases the metabolic rate, speeds up the heart rate, and activates the brain. There is some evidence that caffeine also releases fatty acids and increases cholesterol levels in the blood (134). Coffee drinking also tends to raise the mean blood pressure. Caffeine also interferes with the ability to relax. Too much coffee drinking during pregnancy is claimed to be associated with developmental defects in newborn babies. It is advisable to restrict coffee drinking to two to three cups a day. Children should not be given cola and chocolate together.

TRANQUILIZERS AND SLEEPING PILLS

Tranquilizers or sleeping pills can be valuable medication when used for a short period or during critical circumstances.

If continued for a few weeks, they become ineffective and the dose has to be increased in order to maintain the effect. After four to six months of use, people become dependent on them and abstinence causes physical withdrawal symptoms. They impair the intellectual faculty and driving performance and can be lethal when combined with alcohol.

Many stress control methods, like deep muscle relaxation and meditation, can give similar anxiety-reducing effects without side effects. They are perfectly safe and completely within the control of the individual. They provide deeper, longer lasting relief and allow a fuller appreciation and experience of life's pleasures and pains.

USEFUL STEPS FOR CHANGING HARMFUL HABITS

- Record your current intake.
- Examine the reasons or patterns associated with those habits.
- Decide on alternative methods to meet the need.
- Monitor your progress on a specially devised chart.
- Solve problems which come up during the period of withdrawal without delay, to avoid returning to old habits.
- Do not accept relapse as a final or hopeless situation. Continue to monitor yourself and try again.
- Reward yourself for good efforts.
- Seek social support for encouragement and moral strength.

15

Improving Physical Fitness

Physical exercise is as necessary to life as water, food, and sunlight. It is indispensable if we wish to stay healthy, strong, and agile. There is nothing like physical activity or a game of sport to release tension. Physical health improves our resistance to stress and disease. The human body was designed for the active life our ancestors led, running to catch food and fighting off predators. Modern city life makes none of these demands on the body, and it is not surprising that many people become stiff, flabby, and fat.

You may be tempted to think that as long as you can drive a car or take the bus or train, why walk? If you can take the elevator, why climb stairs? But if you do not exercise, your muscles will atrophy (waste away), your joints will stiffen, your circulation will become sluggish, you will get depressed, and you will become short of breath at the slightest exertion. Premature heart disease is the biggest price to be paid for our sedentary life. There are innumerable reasons for taking regular exercise.

BENEFITS OF EXERCISE

There are many advantages to taking regular exercise. Some of the most important are:

- It prevents coronary heart disease.
- It increases cardiovascular efficiency.
- It reduces high blood pressure.
- It tones up the muscles and improves the figure.
- It helps you to relax.
- It helps you to sleep better.
- It makes you more alert.
- It regulates your appetite.
- It generates vitality and confidence.
- It improves digestion.
- It increases physical strength.
- It keeps the joints supple.
- It encourages and maintains a good, erect posture.
- It improves mental concentration.
- It promotes mental and spiritual development.
- It may improve your intellectual capacity.
- It makes childbearing less painful.
- It lessens the likelihood of sedentary diseases such as rheumatism, arthritis, diabetes, backache, and depression.
- It is known to help asthmatics.
- It increases productivity.
- It balances body and mind.

THE "S" FACTORS: SAFETY, SUPPLENESS, STAMINA, STRENGTH, AND SATISFACTION

Before you embark on any exercise program or sport activity, it is very important to consider the five so-called "S" factors—safety, suppleness, stamina, strength, and satisfaction—

as described on the following pages. This is even more important if you are suffering from coronary artery disease.

Safety

First of all, make sure that you choose a suitable activity for your age and ability. Join classes where you can get expert advice or read books that will give you the relevant background information. You must also have the correct equipment, if equipment is required.

People often have sudden bursts of enthusiasm and want to get fit as quickly as possible, so they exercise hard and long until they are sore all over. This is not only undesirable but could also be dangerous. If you are about to take up an energetic sport which you abandoned years ago, make sure you build up your strength first, concentrating on the areas which are most likely to be strained by your chosen exercise. Go slowly at first and gradually build up over a period of weeks or even months, until you reach your target level. Start off by doing only half the amount of which you think you are capable, and don't compare yourself with others. Always start with some gentle warm-up exercises and take at least five minutes to cool down afterward. If you know that you have high blood pressure, angina, or other heart trouble, consult your doctor about your proposed activity before embarking on it. If you have a minor, temporary illness, such as a cold or influenza, it is best not to exercise until you have recovered. If in doubt, always consult your doctor.

Suppleness

You need to develop the maximum range of movement of your joints, back, and neck, without causing any strain to your muscles, ligaments, or tendons. The more mobile you are, the less likely you are to develop any aches and pains.

Stretch exercises increase your flexibility. It is always important to relax the muscles that you are trying to stretch in order to encourage your maximum stretch and prevent injury.

An easy stretch can be accomplished comfortably when you are completely relaxed. A developmental stretch causes some discomfort but the stretch increases with practice. And a drastic stretch is painful and should not be attempted in case it causes injury.

How Supple Are You? To test your current suppleness, stand on the floor with your legs stretched and try to touch your toes. If you can reach them easily, you are very supple; if you can only reach your ankles, you are quite supple and should work on improving your suppleness; and if you can only reach somewhere between your knees and your ankles, you are not very supple.

Swimming, gymnastics, judo, and dancing are all good forms of exercise for increasing suppleness, as is Yoga, which improves the flexibility of almost every part of the human body.

Stamina

Stamina means staying power, endurance, or the ability to keep going without gasping for breath. The greater your stamina, the better your circulation, so that plenty of vital oxygen is pumped into working muscles. Stamina is also described as aerobic fitness because it ensures that the oxygen you breathe will be used as efficiently as possible. People with greater stamina have a slower, more powerful heartbeat and can cope with more prolonged and strenuous exertion than those with poor stamina. In order to acquire stamina, you must exercise vigorously, for fifteen to twenty minutes, three or four times a week.

Testing Your Stamina. If you can walk up and down two flights of stairs (about twenty steps each flight) fairly briskly, then hold a conversation without getting out of breath, you have good stamina. If you are over 50 you should be able to run in place for two minutes; if you are under 50, you should be able to run for three minutes.

Taking Your Own Pulse. The pulse is the wave of pressure that passes along every artery following a heartbeat. The best way to take your own pulse is in the radial artery at the wrist. Hold one hand palm upward and place the pads of three fingers of the other hand on the groove on the outer side of the wrist—just below the creases—in line with your thumb. You will be able to feel a pulse quite clearly when your fingers are in the right place.

Use a watch with a second hand. Count the number of beats you can feel in fifteen seconds and multiply by four to obtain the rate per minute.

Training Pulse Rates. The chart shown here gives you the recommended range of training pulse rates for various ages up to the age of 60. If you are over 60, you should ask your doctor for guidance. Just as there is a lower limit below which the value of exercise falls off sharply, so there is an upper limit beyond which there is no additional benefit. It is important, in any case, not to exceed the upper limit of the range for your age, because it would put undue strain on your heart.

Age	Recommended training pulse rate
20	140-170
25	135-165
30	130-160
35	125-155
40	120-150
45	115-145
50	110-140
55	105-135
60	100-130

Pulse Rate and Stamina. Your pulse rate is another indication of stamina. It is very easy to learn how to take it. The maximum rate at which a heart can beat is 220 beats per minute, but that rate decreases by one beat for every year of life. To find out your maximum pulse rate, subtract your age from 220. Your pulse rate during exercise—your training pulse rate—should be 70 percent of the maximum rate for your age.

The recommended training pulse rate can also be calculated by subtracting your age from 200, and then subtracting further a handicap of 40 for unfitness (this handicap may be reduced to 20 once you get fitter). For example, if you are 52 and unfit, your training pulse rate should be 200 − 52 (=148) − 40 = 108.

To begin with you can achieve this rate by running in place. Start by doing this gently for thirty seconds, letting your arms hang down by your side and without attempting to lift your knees too high. Gradually build up to five or six minutes, taking your pulse frequently; do not exceed your prescribed rate.

Strength

The stronger the body, the greater its chances of meeting physical demands without undue strain or injury. Strengthening exercises help you to maintain a well-proportioned body and prepare you for sudden physical demands, such as moving furniture. They are also particularly important in preparing you for certain sports, such as skiing.

Although there is always some overlap, it is important to understand that the exercise that increases your aerobic fitness may not necessarily give you strength, and vice versa. Strength is increased by doing a greater amount of work for a shorter time, such as in weight lifting, while stamina is achieved by doing less work for a longer period of time, such as in jogging.

Satisfaction

It is important to enjoy the exercise you do. If you find it boring you won't keep it up, and if you don't practice it regularly you cannot expect any benefits.

It takes fifteen to twenty minutes of vigorous exercise at least three times a week for six weeks before you will notice any significant increase in strength or stamina. The first few sessions may give you nothing more than aching limbs, but once you get into the habit, you will be sufficiently convinced to want to continue with it, and if you were to give it up your body would undoubtedly miss it. If you practice gentle Yoga, you will feel more supple and be aware of a sense of well-being in a matter of days.

Turn your exercise routine into a social event. Jog with a friend, or if you cannot find a regular companion, join an exercise class or sports club. Exercise should be both convenient and enjoyable. Lay out exercise clothes by your bedside in readiness for your morning's jog. If you have opted for indoor exercise, have an illustrated exercise chart on the wall and put on suitable music while you exercise.

WHICH EXERCISE?

There are many recreational sports and activities to choose from. Which one you choose will depend on your inclination, your abilities and disabilities, the state of your heart, the level of your blood pressure, the amount of time you have free, your environment, and the facilities available. Whatever you choose, work out the plan that suits you best and try to stick to it. If you are in any doubt about whether you are able to do the exercise, consult your doctor.

Warm-Up Exercise

Whatever your chosen form of exercise, it is important to warm up before starting any strenuous activity, so that your heart does not have to start working hard suddenly to supply the muscles with the extra oxygen and nutrients needed during exercise, as well as to stretch cold or stiff muscles. These Yoga-based warm-up exercises are gentle, yet effective, initial movements which stretch your muscles and generally loosen you up before you start swimming or jogging, for example.

Neck Rolling. You may exclude this exercise if you have arthritis or if your neck is painful.

1. This exercise can be done while sitting or standing. Start the exercise by slowly rolling your head around to your left.
2. Continue to roll it around to the back and hold it there briefly. Then slowly roll your head around to the right and hold it there briefly.
3. Raise your chin and turn your face to the right, as far as is comfortably possible. Then let your chin fall down onto your chest.

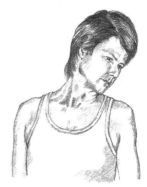

4. Gently push your head down as you slowly move it around to the front again. Repeat the exercise twice.

5. Repeat Steps 1-4 but in the reverse direction. Repeat twice more.

Simple Forward Bending

1. Stand upright with your legs approximately twenty inches apart and your arms by your side. Relax and breathe in.

2. Breathe out and bend forward, letting your arms, head, and trunk just hang down as far as possible.

3. Breathing in, straighten up slowly, keeping your arms, hands, and head relaxed. Straighten your back first and your head last. Stand upright and breathe out. Repeat ten times.

Simple Side Bending

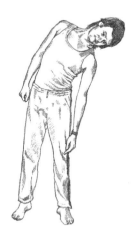

1. Stand upright with your legs approximately twenty inches apart.

2. Breathe in and slowly bend to the left, letting your left hand hang down loosely. Hold for three seconds. Breathe out and slowly straighten up again. Repeat ten times. Carry out the exercise bending to the right ten times.

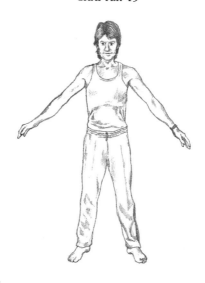

Arm Circling

1. Stand upright with your feet approximately twenty inches apart. Make a slow circling movement with your arms, breathing in as you raise them and breathing out as you lower them.
2. Repeat ten times.

Knee Raising

1. Stand with your feet together and your arms by your sides.
2. Breathe in and gently raise your left knee, grasp your shin, and pull it toward your body, keeping your back straight. Hold for three seconds. Breathe out and return it to the starting position. Repeat with your right leg. Repeat the exercise ten times with each leg.

Exercise Routine

There are numerous keep-fit, aerobic, or Yoga classes available. Join any one of them. Work out a routine for yourself and keep to it. Surely you are worth twenty to thirty minutes, three to five times a week. It is no use choosing exercise you don't enjoy. Some like outdoor activities like golf, tennis, or jogging, while others prefer indoor activities like Yoga or aerobics. Some feel uncomfortable exercising in public, while others need to get away from their own environment and need instruction from a regular teacher in a class. Some like to start the day with exercise, while others may prefer lunchtime or evening sessions after work. Find out what appeals to you and then try to include it in your regular routine.

Jogging

Jogging is a dynamic form of exercise. It is one of the best exercises for attaining cardiovascular fitness. It requires no equipment except a pair of special running shoes to protect your feet and cushion your entire body against the jarring effect of repeated impact. You should lower your heels first, rocking forward on them as when you walk. Don't run on your toes.

Jogging should not be competitive. Just run at a pace that makes you mildly breathless. The steady, easy rhythm helps to ease away tension and leaves you feeling refreshed and revitalized. However, if you have high blood pressure, any heart or circulatory disorder, or arthritis in your legs, do consult your doctor before you start.

Ideally, you should jog every day. If this is not possible, you must jog on alternate days, otherwise you will lose the training effect. If, however, you are not used to it, you should not just rush out one day and start jogging without preparing yourself first. Begin with brisk walks, interspersed with brief jogs. How long you can jog depends on your age and your state of fitness. The most important thing is to build up your schedule gradually, week by week, allowing your heart, lungs, and circulation time to develop stamina. The jogging schedule recommended by the British Health Education Authority is shown below. It gives two programs which give you an idea of how you should build up your own schedule.

When Not to Jog. Avoid jogging immediately after a meal or if you are tired or unwell. Many people find that the best time is early in the morning before breakfast, or after work before supper. If you jog in the dark, wear a reflective jacket or light-colored clothing so that you can easily be seen by motorists. Wear loose-fitting, lightweight clothes that keep you warm but do not make you too hot.

JOGGING SCHEDULES

1. Use this program if you are fairly fit or under 35

Week	Activity
1	Half an hour's brisk walking every day. Walk at every opportunity.
2	Walk 5 mins; jog 30 secs, walk 30 secs, repeat × 10; jog 45 secs, walk 45 secs, repeat × 3; walk 5 mins.
3	Walk 5 mins; jog 1 min, walk 1 min, repeat × 5; walk 5 mins.
4	Walk 2 mins; jog 2 mins, walk 1 min, repeat × 10; walk 2 mins.
5 and after	Walk 1 min; jog 3 mins, walk 1 min, repeat × 5; increase jogging time and cut walking breaks until jogging 20 mins.

2. Use this program if you are unfit or over 35

Week	Activity
1	Half an hour's brisk walking every day. Walk at every opportunity.
2	Walk 5 mins; jog 15 secs, walk 15 secs, repeat × 5; walk 5 mins.
3	Walk 5 mins; jog 30 secs, walk 30 secs, repeat × 3; walk 4 mins; jog 30 secs, walk 30 secs, repeat × 3; walk 5 mins.
4	Walk 5 mins; jog 1 min, walk 1 min, repeat × 2; walk 2 mins, jog 1 min, walk 1 min, repeat × 2; walk 5 mins.
5	Walk 5 mins; jog 1 min, walk 1 min, repeat × 3; walk 5 mins.
6	Walk 2 mins; jog 2 mins, walk 1 min, repeat × 5; walk 5 mins.
7 and after	Increase jogging time and cut down walking breaks until jogging 10-20 mins without break.

Caution

- Consult your doctor if you have high blood pressure, any heart condition, a chest complaint like asthma or bronchitis, arthritis, back pain, or any other problem which you think could be affected if you go jogging.
- Beware of rough ground which could cause injury and, if possible, avoid jogging on hard surfaces, such as roads or pavements, since this jars your spine and other joints. Do not jog up and down hills, as this also has a jarring effect.
- Stop jogging immediately if you feel any chest discomfort.
- Always wear special running shoes. They should have thick soles with good arch support and heel support.

A careless choice of shoes may cause not only discomfort to your feet, but also actual injury to your knees and ankles. Avoid shoes with a plastic lining or high tabs at the back. A good sports shop will be able to advise you.

- Wear comfortable, loose-fitting clothes and avoid synthetic fabrics in which you could get hot and sweaty. Wear a top that can easily be removed once you have warmed up. Wear light-colored or reflective clothing if you jog in the dark.
- Do not jog if you are suffering from any temporary illness, however minor, until you have recovered.
- Do not jog if you feel very tired.
- Watch out for icy roads in winter and avoid jogging if it is foggy.

Walking

For people who are sedentary, who have arthritis or heart problems, or who, for any other reason, consider jogging too strenuous, walking is the safest exercise to embark on. An eight-week schedule in which the activity level is gradually built up is suggested. However, if you don't feel completely satisfied with your progress in a particular week, repeat that week until you can reach the goal with ease. You may wish to know what is a comfortable and what is a brisk walk. A minimum of 60 percent and a maximum of 80 percent of your maximum pulse rate is a good guideline to work on.

However, counting the pulse rate is not the only thing when you exercise. As mentioned earlier, you must enjoy whatever exercise you take up. Jane Fonda's new *Walkout* audio cassette can be very uplifting when you are out and about walking with your personal stereo. She plays several rousing songs, from the "Battle Hymn of the Republic" to "Easy Street"; calls it motivating music; and adds her cheerleading voice. After listening to hundreds of tapes she chose tunes which are everybody's favorites. In the *Walkout Tape I* she starts with a slow cadence—105 steps a minute, with a honky-tonk piano doing "Ragtime Anno 1900." By the time you are into "When Johnny Comes Marching Home," you are up to 114 steps a minute. In half an hour you are back down to 105 steps a minute with "Pomp and Circumstance," so that you cool down before you stop and stretch. She also has *Walkout II* and *Walkout III* tapes, which peak at 126 and 134 steps a minute.

If you tend to stroll while walking, you lose the aerobic fitness schedule, which requires hard striding. With Fonda's music, your mind can wander, but your feet won't let you down, her assistant says. Women can gain double the benefit. They not only improve cardiac fitness but they also help prevent osteoporosis—the condition that occurs when bones become porous and liable to fracture after menopause.

WALKING SCHEDULE

Week 1	Walk at a comfortable pace for 20 minutes.
Week 2	Walk comfortably for 5 minutes, then briskly for 5 minutes. Repeat 3 times.
Week 3	Walk comfortably for 8 minutes, then briskly for 8 minutes. Repeat once more.
Week 4	Walk comfortably for 10 minutes, briskly for 10 minutes. Repeat once again.
Week 5	Walk comfortably for 10 minutes, briskly for 15 minutes and then slowly for 5 minutes.
Week 6	Walk briskly for 20 minutes, then slowly for 10 minutes.
Week 7	Walk briskly for 30 minutes, then slowly for 5 minutes.
Week 8 and after	Walk briskly for 40 minutes, then slowly for 5 minutes.

Indoor Exercise Equipment

When roads are covered with snow or ice, when cold wind is rushing at thirty miles an hour, and when pollution and smog make it unhealthy to be outdoors, there is nothing like indoor exercise equipment, because anything you can do outdoors, you can do indoors with the sophisticated machines now available. In order to ensure that you will not strain your back or ankles it is important to carry out a proper warm-up exercise before going on one of these machines.

Stationary Bikes. These can simulate uphill, downhill, or anything in between. Many of them are fitted with meters which can record your heart rate or the calories burned. You can change pedaling resistance and hence the amount of work you do. They help you improve your aerobic fitness just as well as running or jogging outdoors. All you need is twenty minutes three or four times a week. However, twenty minutes is a long time to sit on a stationary bike, so it is important that you choose one that has a comfortable seat. And if you miss the wind rushing through your hair, you can use wind-load trainers, fan-turbine devices that create wind resistance indoors!

Rowing Machine. While most bicycles work your legs and improve your fitness, they do nothing for your arms. Rowing machines employ arms, legs, shoulders, stomach, and back. There are two varieties available. The hydraulic ones work by pulling the rowing arms against a piston; the one with a cable system works by making your pull spin a flywheel and produce a smooth action similar to rowing on water. This smoothness means less back pain and greater aerobic benefit, since you can build momentum that allows sustained motion. Short individuals may be at a disadvantage with hydraulic rowers, because the handles may force them to pull back too high, caus-ing additional strain on the back.

Treadmills. Although expensive, treadmills remain popu-lar. Ingrid Kristiansen, Norway's woman marathon runner, who set the world record, exercised up to ninety miles a week on one. Not only did she find it safe, but it also meant that she did not have to be away from her husband and her little son. The best machines include incline control so that you can simulate running uphill to raise your heart rate to the de-sired frequency. Nonmotorized treadmills are obviously cheaper but they can cause injury as you are forced to act as the motor and push the belt at the same time as you run.

Strength-Training Devices. In order to increase your mus-cle strength you have to exercise those muscles against resis-tance. None of the machines mentioned so far can overload your muscles. Free weights, rubber tubes, cable body weight machines which use your body weight for resistance, and ma-chines that employ pistons, cables, air, or even water for re-sistance can help you build up your muscles. The resistance machines are safer, though more expensive, than barbells and free weights because they isolate the major groups of muscles while guiding you through motions. Multistation gyms are popular because they offer a greater total body workout al-though they are bulky and expensive. Some fitness experts also point out that moving from one exercise to another doesn't help you to maintain your heart rate long enough to develop maximum fitness.

Most important, before you buy any machine, however, is to consider which machine you are likely to enjoy most because there is no point in buying a machine in a fit of en-thusiasm and then letting it rust because you simply find the exercise boring. Also, don't forget to cool down before you stop exercising. If you suddenly stop, there is a likelihood that a major part of the blood will pool below the waist, reducing the amount going to the brain and making you feel dizzy or even faint.

16

Getting Outside Help

Having identified your stressors and your stress signs, you can use some of the coping strategies I have described so far. However, it is not always easy to cope with stress alone and sometimes we all need to seek the help of others to resolve our problems. For many this is a major barrier. Our tough-minded culture does not allow us to talk to other people easily, particularly to our colleagues or supervisors and sometimes even to our friends and relatives, for fear of being seen as weak or inadequate. So we keep struggling until we are ill, when we feel it is legitimate to go to the doctor. It is important to realize that a lot of unnecessary distress can be avoided and illnesses prevented by enlisting simple help, perhaps just by talking things over with someone.

SOCIAL SUPPORT

Social support depends on the strength and number of supportive social relationships we have. It is increasingly being recognized as useful in reducing stress, protecting health, and enhancing the quality of life.

Definition of Social Support

But what is social support? Like *stress*, the term is generally understood by everyone, but there is confusion when a more accurate definition is required. We know we are supported by our parents in early life and that later on this support is augmented and gradually replaced by support from friends, relatives, spouse, children, and various people at work. But what is social support and how does it work? There are many working definitions but I think the best one is given by James House of the University of Michigan (58). He not only has extensively reviewed the literature on social support but has also carried out some scientific research. He defines social support as having four components:

1. Emotional support, which provides empathy, care, love, trust, or concern. According to researchers, this is the most important component.
2. Instrumental support, which involves behaviors that directly help the person in need, by way of goods or services, for example, someone who can do your gardening when you have strained your back, who will babysit when you are suddenly called elsewhere, or who can lend you money when you have an urgent bill to pay but your check will not clear for another three weeks.
3. Informational support, which provides the person with information which can be used in coping with personal and environmental problems. In contrast to instrumental support, informational support does not help people directly but helps them to help themselves by increasing their resourcefulness. Directing an unemployed person to where he can find a job or a distressed person to where he can get help typifies informational support.

4. Appraisal support is also indirect support, like informational support, except that it relates to self-evaluation by way of social comparison. For example, work supervisor's telling us that we are doing a good job puts us, in our own eyes, above the average. By approving our actions or recognizing them by appropriate means, people can increase our self-esteem and self-worth, which is most important to our sense of well-being.

How Do Ordinary People View Social Support?

When forty single mothers from Canada (43) were asked if there were people who had been helpful to them in dealing with their important personal problems and if so how, a variety of answers were given. Emotional support was identified as having someone to voice concern to, someone who is trustworthy, encouraging, and a good listener, in a relationship that reflects understanding, mutual respect, concern, trust, and intimacy, or as having someone who provides companionship and extended care in times of crisis. The qualities of emotional support enumerated above were reflected in statements like "She'll talk things over with me"; "He seems to have faith in me"; "He listens to me when I talk to him about things"; "She would know what I was saying"; "Some people look down on you, well, she doesn't"; "She expresses her concern for me just by telling me how worried or afraid she is about me"; "She is someone I trust and I knew that it was confidential"; "He is just close to me"; "I've always got her and I really don't feel alone"; "She took the time to be there with me so I didn't have to face it alone"; or "She was with me the whole day."

The kind of support next most important to emotional support turned out to be informational support, and this was indicated by statements like "I am able to tell him what's bugging me and we discuss it." Such discussion often puts things in a new and clear perspective, for example, "making me more aware that I was actually saying other things than I meant to"; other explanations were "He offered suggestions of what I could do"; "He told me to be more assertive"; and "Financially, he put me on to a car mechanic, who gave me a tune-up for less than I would pay in a garage."

Because such a supportive relationship is so often based on respect for the person, he can provide a role model for you, as shown by the following testimony: "Just even watching her and how confident she seems has taught me something." Instrumental support was voiced in examples like "He brought his truck and moved me so I wouldn't have to rent a truck"; "She helped me by talking to the owners and convincing them to wait for the money a while"; and "He'll say, let's go for a drive . . . some little thing to get my mind off it."

Sources of Social Support

A supportive relationship between two individuals certainly involves some cost in terms of time, energy, and sometimes goods or services. It is unlikely that people will always give support altruistically. Giving or receiving social support therefore involves reciprocity and can flourish only in the presence of a stable social relationship.

The sources of support, in decreasing order of priority, are spouse or lover, other family member, friends, people at work, members of religious groups or community organizations, and health care professionals, like general practitioners, counselors, health visitors, or occupational nurses. For stress occurring at work, however, a supportive boss or colleague may be more important than a spouse. Research studies have shown that death rates are lower among people with strong social relationships than among those who live isolated lives (10).

Quality is important as well as quantity. For example, it is not enough to be married; it also matters whether or not the marriage is happy and meets the person's various needs. An adequate measure of social support considers not only the structure of a person's social relationships but also the content, quality, and adequacy of those relationships.

Mechanisms of Social Support

On the basis of growing research evidence, James House suggests that there are three ways in which social support can reduce stress and improve health. The diagram below illustrates these ways.

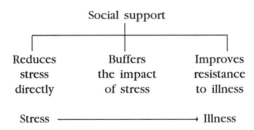

Generally speaking, the greater the stress the greater is the likelihood that one's health will be adversely affected. Social support, House (58) suggests, can help in three possible ways. First, it can directly reduce the level of stress. For example, having supportive co-workers, supervisors, or juniors can reduce interpersonal pressure or tension at work. Such supportive relationships can fulfill the human need for affiliation, approval, and appraisal and thus can make workers more satisfied with their jobs. Second, social support can enhance health and well-being by increasing resistance to illness. It is known that supportive relationships can help instill healthy habits like good nutrition or exercise or can help prevent unhealthy habits like smoking or excessive drinking and can thus generally increase our resistance to stress. The success of Alcoholics Anonymous, Weight Watchers, and other self-help groups is due to this principle. People from all walks of life can meet in such groups and help each other in a way no one else can. No one understands the dilemma better than someone who has been there. Third, and more important, supportive relationships buffer or mitigate the impact of stress on our health and increase a sense of well-being.

Social support therefore has two main effects: it reduces stress regardless of level of health, and it improves health regardless of the level of stress. Thus everyone can benefit from an enhanced level of social support. On the other hand, if a supportive relationship has primarily buffering effects, which counteract or mitigate the adverse impact of stress on health and thus work as moderators of stress, then such a relationship will be of significant value to people with higher levels of stress and will be of lesser or no value to people experiencing little or no stress. For example, social support can mitigate the effect of stressful situations like having a boring job, being unemployed, or having a heavy workload by altering the perception of the situation so that it is seen as less threatening to start with, and then facilitating a defense against such stress by improved coping efforts. For example, an intimate and supportive relationship may put the stress from job dissatisfaction in perspective by helping the person gain a sense of accomplishment and satisfaction outside of work which may wholly or partly compensate for the lack of satisfaction in the work situation.

A man with a supportive family and social network is more adept at finding ways to cope with stress. People in our lives with whom we can talk, who will listen to us, who will encourage us when our confidence seems to be receding, whom we can trust and respect, and to whom we can turn for companionship when lonely are a great source of strength. If, on the other hand, we have no one to turn to or feel a stranger in the community in which we live, we are very vulnerable.

For many, religion provides strong support through its principles and beliefs and through the opportunity of sharing those beliefs with others. Religion can also offer relief from loneliness and a sense of community that helps people feel they are part of something outside themselves. Religious belief itself can be a powerful source of social support in times of stress. The faithful can proceed calmly with their routine, leaving God in charge of their safety and well-being.

Scientific Evidence of the Benefit of Social Support

So far we have intuitively speculated about why social support may reduce stress, improve health, and moderate the impact of stress on health. However, such theories need to be tested. For this we need, first, to make observations on groups of humans or animals exposed to different levels of social support and to study their pattern of health and illness and, second, to experimentally increase social support for one group of people and observe the effect on the health in comparison with the health of a similar group of people with whom no such intervention has taken place.

It has been shown, for example, that a close-knit community of German Protestants living in Nazareth, Pennsylvania, had a much lower rate of coronary heart attack than the rates in nearby non-German communities (16). Similarly, Catholic Americans of Italian origin in Roseto, Pennsylvania, had lower heart attack rates than the people in neighboring communities (132). In a study of 10,000 Israeli civil servants it was found that the incidence of angina in men who perceived their wives as loving and supportive was only half that in those who did not perceive their wives as supportive (86).

The health-sustaining role of a social support system was strongly suggested by Lisa Berkman and Leonard Syme from a study in Alameda County, California, in which 4,700 men and women were followed for nine years (10). The death rate was three times higher in men who were unmarried, who had fewer social contacts with friends and relatives, and who were not church members. Marital status did not make much difference in women, but close relationship patterns and church or social club membership were associated with a lower death rate.

Japan, even though an industrialized country, has the lowest rate of coronary heart disease in the world. However, when Japanese people move to Hawaii, the rate goes up, and when they move to California, it reaches a peak close to the American rate, although not every Japanese-American is affected in the same way. Those Japanese-Americans living in California who maintain their traditional, close-knit social traditions have a lower heart disease rate than Japanese-Americans who have adopted an American or Western way of life. A study from the University of California at Berkeley has shown that this difference among the Japanese living in California cannot be explained by an increase in dietary fat, body weight, blood pressure, smoking, or other established causes of coronary heart disease (79).

How does Japanese social structure protect people from the effect of stress, which takes such a huge toll in terms of premature deaths from coronary artery disease in Western industrialized countries? Scott Matsumoto suggests that the Japanese way of life may be generally more supportive (81). According to him, there is an increasing emphasis on individualism in the West, based on the relative autonomy of the person. In Japan collectivity orientations have been strongly maintained, while there has been a shift from the traditionally hierarchical to an increasingly egalitarian principle. The modern Japanese tend to judge one another rather less as individuals than as representatives of groups. The Japanese value system stresses group welfare and group consensus. The immediate work group is of primary importance. There is a tremendous feeling of in-group solidarity. If asked about his work, a Japanese male will most likely reply by stating the name of his firm rather than his occupation. Once he joins a firm he usually stays there for the rest of his life.

Japanese organizations, in return, show a great deal of paternalism by offering various welfare benefits, exclusively to their own employees, like free medical care, rent-free or low-rent housing, subsidized restaurants and bars, free recreation, and cheaper food and other provisions in company cooperatives. Once hired, an employee is never dismissed except in cases of gross negligence, disobedience, or crime. Seniority as much as competence is important for advancement in wage and rank.

In Japan, Dr. Matsumoto (81) suggests, achievement and mobility are encouraged, but only within the same membership group; there is no motivation to gain admission into a new group: "Only through the intimate group membership, that absorbs his total personality, does the individual find meaning to his existence." Among his fellow employees the Japanese individual can relax, argue, criticize, and be obstinate without endangering relations. When attacked by an outsider, the individual, right or wrong, will have the group's support and backing. There is a greater sense of mutual tolerance and respect among group members. There is also a great deal of socializing among fellow workers after work hours, when they may bathe together or drink together and generally let their defenses down.

Another example of how social support protects health was described by Dr. Roberto Sosa and his colleagues (130) in a study from Guatemala, where it was shown that expectant mothers accompanied by friends had fewer complications than those who were unaccompanied. Such a supportive presence provided emotional and appraisal support. Knowing that someone who cares is there can reassure us and put us in a calm frame of mind. When these others are seen remaining calm in the situation, we are able to reappraise the situation as less threatening. A similar observation about the protective effect of the presence of significant others has been made in animal experiments. In 1950 H. Liddell showed that a young goat isolated in an experimental chamber and subjected to repetitive stress developed experimental neurosis, while its twin in an adjoining chamber, subjected to the same stress, but with the mother goat present, did not (72). However, the presence of others who are likely to make us aware of danger or of our shortcomings can increase our stress. In that situation, ignorance really can be bliss.

In 1977 B. Raphael published a study in which recent widows were randomly assigned to either an intervention group or a control group (111). The intervention group was given a few hours of supportive, nondirective individual counseling in their own homes, while the control group had no such supportive intervention. The results showed that 60 percent of the control group widows suffered a major subsequent health impairment, while less than 25 percent of the intervention group suffered similarly. Belonging to a nonjudgmental, confidential support group directed by peers who have suffered a similar loss is one of the best ways of overcoming loss because it reassures mourners that they are not alone. Such support groups provide people who have lost a loved one with a place where they can share their emotions and pain in a nonthreatening environment, where they can go through that spiritual lesson that we need to celebrate those we love while we can, because they are not ours to keep forever; they are only loaned to us for a while to keep us company on what ultimately seems to be, for each of us, a solitary journey.

There is some evidence to suggest that even pets can provide a buffer against stress and illness. It has been reported that patients were more likely to recover from their heart attacks if they owned a pet or had a satisfactory job to go back to than if they did not. Thus, a social support system which encourages behaviors like loving, touching, caring, and sharing promotes courage, faith, hope, and self-esteem and eventually protects health.

An interesting observation was made at Ohio University, where it was shown that even animals were healthier if they had a support system. A group of investigators studied the effects of a diet high in fat and cholesterol in rabbits. After a predetermined period, the rabbits were sacrificed and certain arteries were examined for evidence of hardening, or what is medically called *atherosclerosis*. In most of the rabbits, the results were as predicted. However, there was a group of rabbits that were far less severely afflicted, and it turned out that the group belonged to an assistant who, in addition to her usual task of feeding the animals and cleaning the cages, had taken them out of the cages and petted, stroked, and talked to them. To make sure that this was not just a coincidence, the investigators carried out another controlled study and showed that petted and stroked rabbits had 60 percent less atherosclerosis! It is a pity that we do not touch and hug our friends and families more often (94).

Social Support in Alleviating Work Stress

The supportive behavior of work supervisors and co-workers can improve both the morale and the productivity of workers and can reduce many forms of organizational stress. It has been shown that as group cohesiveness increases, anxiety over work-related matters decreases.

Planned changes in organizational structure can have the greatest impact on the quality of working life. In the British coal mines, groups of miners traditionally worked together and shared in all aspects of the operation—cutting, drilling, blasting, loading, and extending roof supports. With the introduction of special heavy machines for each of these tasks, each miner became a specialist in one or two operations. The result was diminished job satisfaction, higher absenteeism, and lower productivity. To remedy this situation, researchers from the Tavistock Institute in London constructed a situation in which the old social organization of mining was imposed on the new technological structure, so that a group of workers were given responsibility for a set of tasks and then allowed to decide how to organize their work and share jobs. The result was a lower level of absenteeism, higher productivity, and a reduced level of perceived occupational stress.

In the Volvo automobile assembly plant in Sweden, the assembly process has been similarly designed so that instead of each worker's performing a single task along a continuous conveyor belt, groups work together in a bay on a cluster of assembly tasks. Partly finished cars move from bay to bay, but within each bay a group of workers cooperate in performing a series of tasks by joint decisions. Such collaborative tasks increase group cohesiveness and job satisfaction and reduce stress.

James House (58) and his colleagues at the University of Michigan studied the effects of social support in a large manufacturing plant. They measured, through a questionnaire, how much support each of the workers received from his supervisor, other people at work, spouse, friends, and relatives. Support from supervisor and co-workers moderately reduced all forms of perceived work stress. It was found that outside sources of support, such as from spouse, friends, and relatives, had little or no direct effect on the perception of work stress or direct effect on health, but all the sources of support had buffering effects. Support from the supervisor turned out to be the most important. R. D. Caplan and his colleagues (17) studied over 2,000 male workers from twenty-three different occupations, from physicians to assembly-line workers, and the results were basically the same as those of House and his colleagues. However, they also showed that the benefits of social support are not restricted just to factory workers but are applicable across many occupations.

How to Generate Effective Social Support

In order to use social support to reduce stress and improve health, we need to know how to create and enhance such support where and when necessary. Such knowledge requires understanding of the causes or determinants of social support and how it can be enhanced. Our knowledge is far from complete but enough is known to make a beginning. We can demand or buy support from professional or specialist people whose job it is to give support, such as doctors, counselors, social workers, mental health workers, and clergy; but the informal or natural support relationship between two people, which has the greatest potential for reducing work stress or buffering its impact, is likely to be a reciprocal exchange relationship. Since most beneficial sources of support for reducing work stress differ from those for nonwork stress, they will be considered separately.

Getting Support from People at Work. Since supportive interaction with co-workers is often limited in industrial and office jobs as well as in those jobs which are semiautonomous, like sales and service jobs, work supervisors are considered the primary targets for efforts to enhance work-related social support. The question is: What determines the supportiveness of supervisors? What is it that they do which makes them be perceived as supportive? What causes them to act in a supportive manner? Human relations writer R. Likert (73) describes a supportive supervisor as follows:

> He is supportive, friendly, and helpful rather than hostile . . . genuinely interested in the well-being of subordinates. . . . He sees that each subordinate is well trained for his particular job. He endeavors to help subordinates to be promoted . . . giving them relevant experience and coaching, whenever the opportunity offers. . . . He coaches and assists employees whose performance is be-

low standard. In the case of a subordinate who is clearly misplaced and unable to do his job satisfactorily, he endeavors to find a position well suited to that employee's abilities and arranges to have the employee transferred to it.

However, human relations writers are not quite sure exactly how supervisors can become like this. Many mature adults can be trained in some of these skills. Experience suggests that with appropriate training, paraprofessional or lay counselors can provide as effective counseling as mental health professionals in a number of situations. However, creating supportive supervisory relationships is not simple and they are even more difficult to sustain. One of the most important determinants seems to be what the work organization, especially the higher level of management, advocates, values, and actually rewards. Unfortunately, managerial and organizational support given initially for experimental changes often wanes with time in the face of demands for greater productivity and efficiency (9).

Sustained changes are likely to occur only in the context of broad organizational support for and participation in such changes. Supportive supervision is also more likely to be instituted where the number of subordinates and the nature of the tasks allow the participation of groups of subordinates in planning and organizing work activities.

Trade unions can do a great deal to provide supportive relationships for their members. Union officials are more concerned about the welfare of the workers than employers or supervisors. A shop steward with appropriate training can therefore replace or complement a supervisor as a source of social support. Union bosses with clear commitments are also in a position to effect changes in managerial practices and organizational structure that can facilitate supportive relationships. Employees themselves can be trained to give and receive social support.

Getting Support from People Outside Work. A spouse or partner, close friends, and relatives can be effective sources of social support. Unfortunately, industrialization, urbanization, slum clearance, unemployment, and population growth have meant greater social, cultural, and geographical mobility. As a result, people often have to live away from their kith and kin, in a community of complete strangers. Besides, not all kinds of families and friendship networks are able to provide a similar degree of relevant support. For years both laypeople and scientists have assumed the wife or mother to be the provider of social support to the husband or son. The image of the domestic wife still lingers on. The workers studied by researchers are mainly males and spouse support almost always means wife support. Such sexist attitudes need to be changed in the face of the increased number of women working outside the home. Social support for women by men is just as necessary as support for men by women.

Partners need to be aware of the potential benefit of mutually supportive relationships and to want to exploit it; otherwise the burden of job and family responsibilities may leave little time or energy for sharing and caring. One important requirement for giving and receiving mutual support is the ability to communicate in an empathetic, nonjudgmental, and nondefensive way. To admit unhappiness at work may be difficult for men who like to present a macho image. Sometimes such a sharp line is drawn between work and home that one is hardly ever brought into the territory of the other. However, excessive stress at work may disrupt or weaken the supportive relationships between the worker and his or her family members, thus making family support less available at times when extra support is required. The family life of those who feel unhappy and tense at work is more likely to be characterized by unhappiness, hostility, and tension. Devoting excessive time to work and leaving almost none for the family may also jeopardize family relationships.

Another source of support outside work is professional health care workers. Unfortunately, people seek this support only when work stress has already strained their physical, psychological, or behavioral well-being. There is a great need for both professions and organizations to become involved in preventive work.

In summary, our knowledge of the determinants of social support, both at work and outside of work, is limited in many ways. However, we can and should endeavor to enhance social support at work and try to understand individual as well as organizational motivation and ability to provide such support. Many organizations, especially in the United States and Scandinavia, are increasingly offering stress management courses oriented toward helping individuals. These include relaxation, meditation, exercise, and weight reduction sessions, as well as alcohol and drug abuse programs. They could and should include efforts to improve social support. However, increasing social support on an individual level will be only a drop in the ocean if efforts are not also made to restructure work environments to make them more supportive and less alienating. Social support is not a panacea for all problems and is certainly not a substitute for reducing the level of occupational or other stresses, which should remain a priority.

Training Key People to Be Supportive

Work supervisors, managers, and shop stewards are established channels of authority and communication, and they can serve as important sources of social support if they acquire appropriate skills. The salient points in their training, according to House, are accessibility, an ability to provide an emotional relationship, training to understand the problems of individual workers, a commitment to providing positive help, and use of the resources available strategically to reach the people most in need of support.

Accessibility. Key people must be easily accessible both physically and psychologically. They must ensure that conditions at work facilitate rather than impede free and open communication between workers. Jobs which are highly individualized and do not require cooperation between workers in a group can be physically isolating and nonsupportive. Even when people work in groups, being the only woman or belonging to an ethnic minority can be profoundly socially isolating. Such people are often taken on as a token of social integration or equal opportunity, but they are both exposed to unique work stresses and largely cut off from others who would be likely to understand and empathize with their situation. Key people must be aware of this possibility and must be prepared to foster women's or minority workers' "networks" within organizations. These networks also facilitate communication and support between majority and minority groups.

Training People to Provide Support. Key people must be trained to be supportive. Merely telling them to be helpful or supportive is not only not helpful but may also be counterproductive. Most people need some training in the four components of social support mentioned earlier; emotional support is the most important skill and also the most difficult to transmit. Emotionally sustaining behavior is not just cheering people up; it requires empathic listening to others' problems with expressions of positive regard and the ability to create a feeling of trust and intimacy. Key people must necessarily be good communicators. In a review of good supervisors, W. C. Redding (112) listed the following qualities:

- The better supervisors tend to be more "communication-minded"; for example, they enjoy talking and speaking up in meetings; they are able to explain instructions and policies; they enjoy conversing with subordinates.
- The better supervisors tend to be willing, empathic listeners; they respond with understanding to so-called silly questions from employees; they will listen to suggestions and complaints with an attitude of fair consideration and willingness to take appropriate action.
- The better supervisors tend to "ask" or "persuade" in preference to "telling" or "demanding."
- The better supervisors tend to be sensitive to the feelings and ego defense needs of their subordinates; for example, they are careful to reprimand in private rather than in public.
- The better supervisors tend to be more open in their passing along of information; they are in favor of giving advance notice of impending changes, and of explaining the reasons behind policies and regulations.

Rewards and Reinforcement. Simple acquisition of the skills of listening, communication, and caring is not enough if they are not used continuously and properly rewarded or reinforced. Traditionally, in productivity-oriented Western industries dominated by macho men, empathy, consideration, and sensitivity are thought to be soft, nonproductive, feminine options which work against efficiency. This is wrong. The commitment of higher-level management as well as of workers to group affiliation and social bonding in Japan have amply demonstrated that they are likely to increase, not decrease, productivity. An emphasis on material gain alone is bound to fail. Therefore it is important that organizations and unions not only encourage and train their key people to provide social support but also that such efforts on the part of the key people be properly acknowledged and rewarded.

Helping Others to Help Yourself

There are some indications that helping others improves the health of those who lend the helping hand. The benefits of altruism, long preached by moralists, are now being confirmed scientifically. Members of Alcoholics Anonymous learned long ago that helping others can also help them to beat the bottle. Recovering alcoholics are expected to support others who are struggling to free themselves of their addiction. They find that this helping role, difficult though it may be, creates a feeling of inner strength that helps them overcome their own problem.

James House (58) and his colleagues from University of Michigan found that regular volunteer work, more than anything else, dramatically increased the life expectancy of men. Robert Ornstein and David Sobel, the authors of *The Healing Brain* (96), suggest that the brain's primary function is not to think but to protect the body from illness and that it cannot do its job without contact with other people. They say, "Evolution has less regard for the individual than for the survival of the species. Our brain may have evolved to protect our health so that we could contribute to the survival of the kind."

Hans Selye, in his classic book *The Stress of Life* (122), coined the phrase "altruistic egotism" to describe this selfish need to help others. With regard to how it works, he suggested that by doing good for people, we inspire their gratitude and warmth and that this warmth protects us from the stress of life. Scientists are also finding that helping others can be good for the nervous system and immune system, which are intimately connected. The nerve cells connect the brain with the parts of the body—the bone marrow and spleen that produce the immune system cells necessary to fight off infection and cancer cells. Married women seem to have better immune function than unmarried or divorced women, and happily married women have the healthiest immune function of all. It has been said that virtue, like gold, is stronger when alloyed with a baser metal. It is suggested that we need to develop plenty of virtuous strength even if at times a little enlightened selfishness is required to drive us.

Review Your Social Network: Excercise

Source	Name of person	Level of satisfaction (1 = low; 2 = medium; 3 = high)
1. Spouse/partner	_____	_____
2. Mother/father	_____	_____
3. Brother/sister	_____	_____
	_____	_____
	_____	_____
4. Close friend(s)	_____	_____
	_____	_____
5. Other relatives	_____	_____
	_____	_____
6. Work associates	_____	_____
	_____	_____
	_____	_____
7. People with common interests (e.g., member of club or organization)	_____	_____
	_____	_____
	_____	_____
	_____	_____
8. Church group	_____	_____
	_____	_____
9. Counselor/mentor	_____	_____
	_____	_____
10. Community leader	_____	_____
11. Financial adviser	_____	_____
12. Other significant person(s)	_____	_____
	_____	_____
	_____	_____

13. Person who shows
    sympathy for or
    empathy with you

14. Person who can
    advise, suggest, direct,
    and generally add to
    your resourcefulness

15. Person who approves
    of you

16. Person who is
    prepared to help
    more tangibly (e.g.,
    lend you money

17. A pet

Total score

The size of present support system: _____

The quality of present support system: _____

    1 = less than adequate

    2 = about right

    3 = more than necessary

Identify three people with whom you would like to establish or
improve your relationship

1. _____

2. _____

3. _____

PROFESSIONAL HELP

Many of us know people to whom we can go in times
of crisis, not because they have special qualifications but because they seem to listen with warmth and understanding.
Many work organizations have such people who are specially
trained in counseling. These are welfare officers as well as

training and development officers. They can listen objectively, and such listening often helps in solving problems. Merely answering their probing questions may suddenly clarify the issues for you and you may quickly find a solution yourself. If the problem is beyond their scope they are often in a position to refer you to someone who can help you. Even if you think that your manager, your supervisor, or even your boss is not trained in counseling, it may be worth going to him and discussing your problem because, contrary to some people's belief, he is interested in your health and may be in a position to offer you a constructive solution. In addition, your doctor and many other counseling and professional organizations are ready to help and it is up to you how much you are prepared to do for your own health. A parable retold below shows that even God can't help unless you help yourself (62):

> Once upon a time it rained so much that an entire village was flooded. Many houses were destroyed and there was water everywhere. Rescuers came and helped villagers to safe places but there was a man who refused to be rescued. He was an honest, hard-working, religious man who prayed regularly and never did anything wrong. He climbed on to the roof of his house and waited there, believing that God would save him. People threw pieces of logs and finally a boat came, but he refused to come down, saying, "God will help me." The rains continued, the flood got worse and the man was drowned. In heaven, he complained to God, "Why didn't you help me? I was your staunch devotee and you did not come to my rescue." God answered, "I sent you three rafts and a boat and you refused to be saved." For some you can never do enough.

Saving health is more important than saving face, so please do not hesitate to go to the appropriate people for help. The role of voluntary organizations or self-help groups has already been mentioned.

17

Coping with People Who Create Stress in Others

Coping with difficult people is the commonest source of stress for many. The term *people poisoning* is sometimes applied to stress caused by such people. We may even call them *stress generators* or *stress carriers*, as they are often the people who give others stress without suffering from it themselves. Have you come across any of the following?

- An indecisive, vacillating boss
- An irritating, "bite-your-head-off" supervisor
- A junior who agrees with everything but does nothing
- An unhelpful, "I-don't-want-to-know-about-it" colleague
- Hostile customers
- A moaning and groaning secretary
- An intransigent manager

If so, maybe you can be helped. Remember, we are not talking about people who occasionally fly off the handle. We can all sometimes drag our feet or take on things that are beyond our capacity. What we are concerned about are those who frustrate or demoralize us.

In order to cope with these stress carriers effectively, we need to understand the patterns of their behavior which transmit stress. Obviously, an individual's behavior does not always fall into clearly defined types and there is a considerable overlap. In order to simplify a very complex subject, the following classification was used by Dr. Robert Bramson (12), based on his extensive experience as a long-standing management consultant. He says there are basically seven types of stress carriers: hostile aggressives, complainers, silent unresponsives, superagreeables, pessimists, know-it-all experts, and indecisive stallers. Their characteristics and ways of coping with each type, based on Dr. Bramson's experience, are summarized below.

HOSTILE AGGRESSIVES

People in this category have a tendency to bully or overwhelm you with powerful speeches. They ridicule or humiliate you by their remarks, which often contain corrosive or obscene phrases. Sometimes they employ more subtle methods and make hostile jokes or sarcastic remarks. They have a tendency to criticize you personally, not your mistakes. With such treatment they confuse, frighten, or frustrate you and leave you either in tears or raging mad.

When such negative emotions take over, you can lose your power of rational thinking. They get irritated because you cannot see as clearly as they can. If they don't get their own way, they sometimes explode and adopt tantrumlike behavior, during which they will make fearsome attacks with all the rage and fury they can command, throw objects, or even strike a blow. Such eruptive behavior, barely under control, has become a part of their repertoire, probably there since childhood.

Sometimes they use a more covert method, especially if you are in a dominating position. For example, if they disagree with you, they will wait until your back is turned and they will make a thumbs-down sign or whisper to other people, "What a boring meeting" or "How dull can a person get?"

Coping Methods

The following are some of the strategies you can use to cope with hostile aggressives (12).

Stand Up for Yourself. Don't let them push you around. You must try to say something of an assertive nature like "Hang on, I've got something to say to you" or "You've got to hear me out—I, too, have a point." You may have to give them some time to calm down before you can get your word in. Sometimes you can get their attention if you drop a pencil or book or stand up or sit down. Use whatever ploy is necessary to interrupt them, without worrying about being polite. If possible get them to sit down, as people are less aggressive when sitting down.

Express Your Opinion. Use self-assertive phrases, like "In my opinion . . ." or "I disagree . . ." or "I believe." Do not, however, shout back, as a shouting match is not likely to be helpful.

Avoid a Collision Course. Don't try to win. Even if you win a battle, you are sure to lose the war. One defeat is not likely to cure such expert hostile aggressives of their affliction. If the situation gets very hot and rational conversation becomes impossible, suggest a break. If your suggestion is completely ignored, you can leave the scene, saying that you will be back later.

Accept Their Friendship. When a hostile aggressive knows that you won the point by standing up for your opinion, he may suddenly become friendly and extend his hand or offer to buy you a drink. If so, accept without hesitation. It is better to have such a person as your friend than as an enemy.

In Case of Covert Attacks. Try to uncover the attack and seek opinions from the rest of the group. If the others don't agree with him, he will stop his tactics. Whatever you do, don't give him the platform by saying, "All right, you tell me how you would do it better." This is exactly what he wants, so that he can weaken your leadership. The best thing is to prevent such attacks by regular meetings where people are given an opportunity to air their grievances.

COMPLAINERS

These are people who constantly whine and complain about things but who never try anything to solve the problems they are complaining about. They usually approach your desk and sit down. Their long-winded sentences are connected with *ands* and *buts* as they self-righteously accuse and blame others. They don't offend you like the hostile aggressives but they can be exhausting and irksome. Don't confuse them with those emotional people who occasionally need your shoulder to cry on. The moaners are completely in control of their emotions and know exactly what should be done and who should be doing it. Pointing these things out to you makes them feel morally right and innocent. In fact, they often point out real problems, but the way they do it can make you defensive.

Coping Methods

The following are some of the strategies you can use to deal with these moaners and groaners (12).

Take Them Seriously. They continue with their rituals because they themselves feel powerless to do anything, and because of their nature nobody takes them seriously enough to solve the problems they are pointing out. To break the vicious circle, you need to listen to them attentively. Once you have the gist of the problem, however, do interrupt; otherwise their complaints may never end. Acknowledge what they are saying by paraphrasing, without agreeing or defending, as agreeing makes them convinced that they were right all along.

Take Steps to Solve the Problem. In order to get to the bottom of the problem ask searching questions like "When, where, and how?" Don't ask why questions, or you will be subjected to long-winded explanations. If they still go back to their former course, interrupt, acknowledge, and start again.

Delegate a Task. Ask them to gather relevant information. If necessary, ask them to put it in writing. However, don't use this tactic just to sweep the matter under the carpet. Be serious about solving the problem. Give a time limit and follow the problem up.

Stop Further Interaction. In spite of your trying earnestly to solve the problem, if the person continues to moan and groan, ask how he wants to end the discussion, which is not taking you anywhere.

SILENT UNRESPONSIVES

People who maintain silence after you have given a well-prepared sales speech or have made a good presentation, when you are expecting comments, questions, or discussion, can be unnerving. You may have some reservations about one of your juniors but he remains silent to any questions you ask. It is difficult to get anywhere with these people. They are different from those thoughtful people who speak only when necessary. The silent unresponsives purposely remain silent. They use this ploy for a multitude of reasons—to avoid telling a lie, to hide the truth, to humiliate you, as a form of predetermined aggression, or as a spiteful refusal to cooperate. It is difficult to understand why they won't talk. How can you read their minds? If they persist in their behavior the only way you can obtain a clue is from nonverbal communication.

People use a variety of finger, arm, and hand gestures, body stance, facial expressions, and other mannerisms which can sometimes convey powerful messages. I recommend Desmond Morris's book *Manwatching*, which is a fascinating guide to gestures people make when confronted with conflicts or tension, leadership issues or boredom (92). With gestures, people can thank you or abuse you, show humility or hostility.

Coping Methods

The following are some of the strategies you can use to cope with silent unresponsives (12).

Ask Open-Ended Questions. Don't ask questions that can be answered with yes or no. Instead of asking, "Do you agree?" ask, for example, "What is your reaction?"

Remain Silent Until They Answer. When people don't say anything, we find silence uncomfortable and there is a tendency to butt in and fill the gap with our own conversation. If you want these silent people to answer your question, avoid the temptation. Instead, look straight into their eyes and wait patiently, with an expectant expression.

Restart If Necessary. If you cannot break the ice, even after a long silence, it is time for a fresh start. Comment that you were expecting them to say something. Ask what the problem is. What ideas are going through their minds? What makes it so difficult to talk? Again wait silently, expectantly, with a friendly expression.

Allow Sufficient Time. If you are familiar with the tendency of these people, make sure that you have allowed sufficient time for their slow reactions. If they remain silent until the end of your time limit, don't end the issue by saying, for example, "Thank you for coming." Make another appointment and follow up. Sometimes they may say irrelevant things. Let them say them because at least it is a start. Remain silent until they come to the point.

As a Last Resort, Proceed on Your Own. Sometimes you will fail to get any answer despite your patient attempts. You may still, however, get a last-ditch response by putting in writing something like, "I assume from your silence that you agree with what I said." If they don't agree with you, they will have to respond. If they still don't respond, you will be justified in taking whatever steps are necessary.

SUPERAGREEABLES

As the name suggests, these are people who agree with everything you say. Unfortunately, they fail to produce. They agree because they have an incredible need to be loved and liked by everybody all the time. They are outgoing, often funny, and pleasant people. They are sincere and supportive, but despite their willingness, they are incapable of delivering the promised goods. They agree to everything you say because otherwise they fear your disapproval or loss of regard. Rather than jeopardize your friendship, they make unrealistic promises and commitments which they are not in a position to fulfill.

Coping Methods

The following are some of the strategies you can use to cope with these otherwise wonderful people (17).

Encourage Honesty. Be friendly and personal if you can. Put them at ease by saying, for example, "Don't be frightened of giving me your honest opinion." If they look tense, talk about other things like their family or a television program. Once they feel accepted they are more likely to be truthful.

Stop Them from Making Unrealistic Promises. If they start to make commitments which you know to be unreasonable, make realistic counteroffers. For example, give them a week to prepare a project instead of letting them promise to have it ready by tomorrow. Make compromises instead of holding them to their word because they will otherwise make even more unrealistic promises and you won't resolve the problem.

Listen to Their Humor. They often use humor as a double-edged sword to get over a conflict of telling the truth, or to distort it out of all proportion to avoid your displeasure.

Thus they start out by telling you the truth wrapped up in humor. If they see any sign of anger or hurt in you they can easily change the story. If, on the other hand, they see signs of your acceptance, they will proceed with the truth.

PESSIMISTS OR NEGATIVISTS

These are people who respond to other people's constructive suggestions by saying things like, "It won't work"; "We have tried it before and it flopped"; and "It's no use trying." They do not offer alternative suggestions either. They just do not think that there is any possible solution. They say this with such conviction that you begin to believe it. These people can have a very depressing and demoralizing effect on group members, as they shoot down every alternative suggestion or creative idea. Usually in our past we have had a failure or a ruined plan, and so deep down in all of us there is a potential for despair. These pessimists succeed in bringing it out. They are often competent people who argue with such rationality that it is very easy to feel defeated. They don't mean to drag us down, but because of their past failures, they have come to believe that these outside forces are absolute, immutable barriers.

Coping Methods

The following are some of the strategies which you can use to cope with pessimists (12).

Don't Get Drawn In. Be aware of your potential for despair. As soon as you begin to hear anything like "It's impossible, they will never let us do it," you should hear bells ringing, telling you to watch out for depression.

Remain Optimistic. If you want to prevent the entire group's being dragged down, make encouraging statements based on your past successful experience. Try to instill hope and faith in others by saying something like "I am sure there is a way out" or "We must be able to work something out."

Don't Argue or Rush into Proposing a Solution. Arguing to prove pessimists wrong is a waste of time. Besides, they may be right. Ask what is the worst that can happen. That way you are at least preparing for the eventuality. Avoid the temptation of proposing a solution which can be shot down by negativists. Instead, ask searching questions to pinpoint the problem. Once they become intrigued by the task of untangling the problem, they will be off their guard, and a solution can easily be introduced without its being given undue prominence.

Use Negativism Constructively. Even pessimists can be useful sometimes in counterbalancing your unrealistic optimism. Once you understand them and separate hopelessness from the substance of their negative comments, they may be worth heeding. Their caution at least prepares you for a fallback position if, as they warned, your plan does fail.

As a Last Resort, Go on Your Own. If everything fails and a pessimist succeeds in depressing the entire group, you have no choice but to say something like "I think it's worth trying. Would anyone join me? I can use all the help I can get." It will split up the group but there is no alternative.

KNOW-IT-ALL EXPERTS

There are basically two types of know-it-all experts. Bramson calls them bulldozers and balloons (12). The first do know what they are talking about, while the latter do not.

Bulldozers

Bulldozers want you to do things their way and according to their time schedule. They don't want your suggestions, facts, or figures. As the name implies, they are accurate thinkers, thorough planners, and highly productive people who are capable of executing plans despite obstacles. They have powerful personalities and great self-sustaining qualities. They don't believe in luck and think that what they get is entirely due to their own efforts. They are absolutely certain of themselves, and with that conviction and belief, beyond any reasonable doubt, they make you feel very small. They bring out resentment and self-defensive behavior in their associates by dismissing their ideas and suggestions as unimportant or irrelevant.

Coping Methods

The following are some of the strategies you can use (12).

Prepare Yourself Thoroughly. Make sure that you have done adequate homework and checked all your facts and figures. If there is a small discrepancy in your calculations, your entire plan will be dismissed.

Listen and Acknowledge. Pay attention to what they are saying. Acknowledge it by paraphrasing the gist of what they are saying. Acknowledge their expertise and competence.

Question, but Don't Confront. Clarify the details of their plans or suggestions by all means, and how these will stand up in the long run, but do not attack the competence of these people. Avoid becoming a counterexpert. If possible, suggest putting off the decision for a while so that you can have a chance to reflect on their ideas, at the same time requesting them to look at your plans.

Let Them Be the Expert. If they are determined to carry through their plans, there is no point in digging in your heels. Instead, you should let these superior beings be the experts and should even offer to help them with their plans. That way there won't be bitterness, tension, or undue depression.

Balloons

These are people who read a magazine article and become instant experts on the subject. However, they talk with such authority and conviction that unless you know them from previous experience you may find it difficult to differentiate them from bulldozers. In their overwhelming desire to be respected and admired, their supposition becomes reality and the distinction between speculation and wisdom becomes blurred. Unfortunately, they don't even regret leading people astray. If you suffer as a result of their advice, they will feel it is your fault as you should have taken responsibility yourself for checking the details.

Coping Methods

The following are some strategies you can use.

Don't Take Them Seriously. Balloons are only a minor irritation once you are familiar with their lack of depth, so just sit back and let them pontificate.

Provide a Face-Saving Way Out. Don't try to confront them about their lack of knowledge as confrontation is likely to paralyze them. If loss of face becomes apparent, they may resort to primitive behavior. If you must confront them, at least do it in private and not in front of others.

INDECISIVE STALLERS

These are pleasant people who are very helpful and supportive but postpone making decisions week after week. If you depend on them to forward your suggestions to a higher authority or comment on your project or the papers you have worked so hard on, there is nothing more frustrating than to find that those on whom you depend can't make up their minds. This behavior "works" as far as they are concerned because most decisions, if not made, soon become irrelevant. They want to be helpful, but in their conflict between wanting to be honest and not wanting to hurt anyone, they avoid making decisions.

Coping Methods

The following are some of the strategies you can use, as stallers are not otherwise likely to be candid (12).

Make Honesty Nonthreatening. Tell them that you can cope with honest answers, criticisms, or suggestions for improvement. Their gestures, indirect needs, and hesitations may give you some clue to where the problem lies. Gently ask the reason for their conflict or reservation. The reservation may be about you.

Help Them with Problem-Solving Steps. If the source of the problem is you, acknowledge your weakness or deficiency and directly request help. You can state your plan descriptively and undefensively. Offer to sacrifice something from your plan to see if the new plan will be acceptable. If possible, suggest how your plan is likely to improve the quality of life of other people.

Suggest Rank-Ordering Alternatives. Stallers have difficulty in choosing between two alternatives. If there are six alternatives they will be paralyzed. Suggesting rank ordering makes it easier to say to someone that their plan came in second.

Maintain Support or Control, but Don't Overload. If you slacken, once a decision has been made, stallers may revert to their previous state of indecision. If possible, keep control in your hands. If not, see that decisions are acted on as quickly as possible—without applying undue pressure. Watch for signs of overload. If they start yawning, turning pages, or showing other signs of tension, do not pursue the matter further at that point, but make a strategic withdrawal, saying something like "I will see you later." Otherwise, in a tense state, they may make a hasty decision which they will refuse to change.

GENERAL ADVICE

- Avoid these stress generators if at all possible. If this is not possible, accept that they are difficult people.
- Make plans based on the strategies given. Since no two moaners or know-it-all experts are exactly the same, you will have to take into consideration your own personal experience of them before making the final plan.
- Rehearse your plan adequately. Try to tackle minor problems first, probably with your juniors or peers, before tackling a major problem or people in very high positions. Once you have learned to cope effectively with modestly difficult people and have gained suffi-

cient confidence, you can cope with more difficult people later.

- Execute your plan. Even if you are not 100 percent successful, don't despair. Compliment yourself on whatever success you have. In case of complete failure, have a fallback position ready. With repeated efforts you are bound to succeed.
- Monitor the effectiveness of your plan. Modify the plan if necessary and reexecute it.

Bibliography

1. Alexander, Franz. (1939). Emotional factors in essential hypertension: Presentation of tentative hypothesis. *Psychosomatic Medicine*, 1: 173-179

1a. Antonovsky, A., Maoz, B., Dowty, N., and Wijsenbeek, H. (1971). Twenty-five years later. *Social Psychiatry*, 6: 186-193.

2. Atkinson, Holly. (1987). *Women and Fatigue*. New York: Pocket Books.

3. Baker, L. J., Dearborn, M., Hastings, J. E., and Hamberger, K. (1984). Type A behaviour in women: A review. *Health Psychology*, 3: 477-497.

4. Barefoot, J. C., Dahlstrom, G., and Williams, R. B. (1983). Hostility, CHD incidence and total mortality: A 25-year follow-up study of 255 physicians. *Psychosomatic Medicine*, 45: 59-63.

5. Bartrop, R. W., Luckhurst, L., Kiloh, L. G., and Penny, R. (1977). Depressed lymphocyte function after bereavement. *Lancet*, 1: 834-836.

6. Belgian-French Pooling Project. (1984). Assessment of Type A behaviour by the Bortner scale and ischemic heart disease. *European Heart Journal*, 5: 440-444.

7. Bengtsson, C., Hällstrom, T., and Tiblin, G. (1973). Social factors, stress experience and personality traits. In women with ischemic heart disease compared to population sample of women. *Acta Medica Scandinavica*, 549: 82-92.

8. Benson, Herbert. (1975). *The Relaxation Response*. New York: Morrow.

9. Berg, I., Freedman, M., and Freeman, M. (1978). *Managers and Work Reform: A Limited Engagement*. New York: Free Press.

10. Berkman, Lisa, and Syme, Leonard. (1979). Social networks, host resistance and mortality: A nine-year follow-up of Alameda County residents. *American Journal of Epidemiology*, 109: 186-204.

11. Bloom, Lynn Z., Coburn, Karen, and Pearlman, Joan. (1975). *The New Assertive Woman*. New York: Dell.

12. Bramson, Robert M. (1981). *Coping with Difficult People*. New York: Ballantine Books.

13. Brickman, Harry R. (1971). Mental health and social change: An ecological perspective. In H. P. Dreitzel (Ed.), *The Social Organization of Health*. New York: Macmillan.

14. Brown, G. W. Experiences of discharged chronic schizophrenic patients in various types of living groups. *Millbank Memorial Fund Quarterly*, 37: 105-131.

15. Brown, G. W., and Harris, T. (1978). *Social Origins of Depression—A Study of Psychiatric Disorders in Women*. London: Tavistock.

16. Bruhn, J. G., Wolf, S., Lynn, T., Bird, H., and Chandler, B. (1968). Social aspect of coronary heart disease in a Pennsylvania German community. *Social Science and Medicine*, 2: 615-626.

16a. Cannon, W. B. (1963). *The Wisdom of the Body*. New York: W. N. Norton.

17. Caplan, R. D., Cobb, S., French, J. R. P., Harrison, R. V., and Pinneau, S. R. (1975). *Job Demands and Worker Health*. HEW Publication No. (NIOSH) 75-160, Washington, D.C., U.S. Department of Health, Education and Welfare.

18. Carmen, E., Russo, N., Miller, F., and Baker, J. (1981). Inequality and women's mental health: An overview. *American Journal of Psychiatry*, 138: 1321-1325.

19. Carnegie, Dale. (1985). *How to Win Friends and Influence People*. New York: Pocket Books.

20. Cohen, J. B., and Reed, D. (1984). The Type A behaviour pattern and coronary heart disease risk among Japanese men in Hawaii. *Journal of Behavioural Medicine*, 8: 343-352.

21. Cole, Lamont C. (1971). Playing Russian roulette with biogeochemical cycles. In H. P. Dreitzel (Ed.), *The Social Organization of Health*. New York: Macmillan.

22. Cottington, E. M., Matthews, K. A., Talbot, E., and Kuller, L. H. (1980). Environmental events preceding sudden death in women. *Psychosomatic Medicine*, 42: 567-573.

23. Cox, Tom. (1978). *Stress*. London: Macmillan.

24. Cousins, Norman. (1979). *Anatomy of an Illness*. New York: Bantam Books.

25. Dossey, Larry. (1982). *Space, Time and Medicine*. Boulder and London: Shambhala.

26. Dembroski, T. M., MacDougall, J. M., Williams, R. B., Haney, T. L., and Blumenthal, J. A. (1985). Components of Type A hostility and anger in

relationship to angiographic findings. *Psychosomatic Medicine*, 47: 219-233.

27. Dreitzel, Hans Peter. (1971). *The Social Organization of Health*. New York: Macmillan.

28. Dunbar, H. F. (1943). *Psychosomatic Diagnosis*. New York: Hoeber.

29. Eaker, E. D., Haynes, S. G., and Feinleib, M. (1983). Spouse behavior and coronary heart disease in men: Prospective results from the Framingham Heart Study. *American Journal of Epidemiology*, 118: 23-41.

30. Eastman, Peggy. (1987). Sudden death: Notes on a journey through grief. *New Age Journal*, July/August, 16-20.

31. Eliot, R. S., and Breo, D. L. (1985). *Is It Worth Dying For?* New York: Bantam Books.

32. Engel, G. L. (1955). Studies in ulcerative colitis: The nature of the psychological process. *American Journal of Medicine*, 19: 231.

33. Engel, G. L. (1971). Sudden and rapid death during psychological stress: Folklore and folk wisdom. *Annals of Internal Medicine*, 74: 771-782.

34. Eyton, Audrey. (1982). *The F-Plan Diet*. Harmondsworth, England: Penguin.

35. Frankenhaeuser, Marianne. (1986). A psychological framework for research on human stress and coping. In M. F. Appley and R. Trumbull (Eds.), *Dynamics of Stress*. New York: Plenum Press.

36. Friedman, Meyer, and Rosenman, Ray. (1974). *Type A Behavior and Your Heart*. New York: Knopf.

37. Friedman, M., Rosenman, R., and Carroll, V. (1958). Changes in serum cholesterol and blood clotting in men subjected to cyclic variation of occupational stress. *Circulation*, 17: 852-861.

37a. Friedman, M., Thoresen, C. E., Gill, J. J., *et al.* (1986). Alteration of Type A behavior and its effect on cardiac recurrences in post-myocardial infarction patients: Summary results of the Recurrent Coronary Prevention Project. *American Heart Journal*, 112: 653-665.

38. Friedman, Meyer, and Ulmer, Diane. (1984). *Treating Type A Behavior and Your Heart*. New York: Fawcett Crest Books.

39. Gawain, Shakti. (1982). *Creative Visualization*. New York: Bantam Books.

40. Gillett, R. (1987). *Overcoming Depression*. London: Dorling Kindersley.

41. Glass, David C. (1977). *Behaviour Patterns, Stress and Coronary Disease*. Hillsdale, NJ: Erlbaum.

42. Glass, D. C., Krakoff, L. R., Contrada, R., Hilton, W. F., Kehoe, K., Mannucci, E. G., Collins, C., Snow, B., and Elting, B. (1980). Effect of harassment and competition upon cardiovascular and catecholamine responses in Type A and B individuals. *Psychophysiology*, 17: 453-463.

43. Gottlieb, B. H. (1978). The development and application of a classification scheme of informal helping behaviours. *Canadian Medical Journal of Science*, 10(2): 105-115.

44. Graham, M. H., Douglas, R. M., and Ryan, P. (1986). Stress and acute respiratory infection. *American Journal of Epidemiology*, 124: 389-401.

45. Groen, J. J. (1975). The measurement of emotion and arousal in the clinical physiological laboratory and in medical practice. In L. Levi (Ed.), *Emotions: Their Parameters and Measurement*. New York: Raven Press.

46. Guilleminault, C. and Dement, W. C. (1978). *Sleep Apnoea Syndromes*. New York: Alan R. Liss.

47. Hales, D., and Hales, R. B. (1986). Alcohol: Better than we thought. *American Health*, December, 38-43.

48. Hall, G. S. (1899). A study of anger. *American Journal of Psychology*, 10: 516-591.

49. Harburg, E., Blakelock, E. H., and Roeper, P. J. (1979). Resentful and reflective coping with arbitrary authority and blood pressure: Detroit. *Psychosomatic Medicine*, 41: 189-202.

50. Haynes, S. (1984). Type A behaviour, employment status and coronary heart disease in women. *Behavioural Medicine Update*, 6: 15.

51. Haynes, S., and Feinleib, M. (1980). Women, work and coronary heart disease: Prospective findings from the Framingham Heart Study. *American Journal of Public Health*, 70: 133-141.

52. Haynes, S., Feinleib, M., and Kannel, W. B. (1980). The relationship of psychosocial factors to coronary heart disease of the Framingham study: III. Eight year incidence of coronary heart disease. *American Journal of Epidemiology*, 3: 37-58.

53. Hewitt, James. (1978). *Meditation, Teach Yourself Books*. London: Hodder & Stoughton.

54. Hinkle, Laurence E., and Plummer, Norman. (1952). Life stress and industrial absenteeism. *Industrial Medicine and Surgery*, 21: 365-375.

55. Holmes, T. A. (1956). Multi-discipline studies in tuberculosis. In M. Sparer (Ed.), *Personality, Stress and Tuberculosis*. New York: International Universities Press.

56. Holmes, T. A., and Masuda, M. (1973). Life change and illness susceptibility, separation and depression. *Journal of American Association for the Advancement of Science*, 161-186.

57. Holmes, T. A., and Rahe, R. H. (1967). The Social Readjustment Rating Scale. *Journal of Psychosomatic Research*, 11: 213-218.

58. House, James. (1981). *Work, Stress and Social Support*. New York: Addison-Wesley.

59. Hurley, R. (1971). *The Health Crisis of the Poor in the Social Organisation of Health*. New York: MacMillan.

60. Jacobson, Edmund. (1976). *You Must Relax*. London: Souvenir Press.

61. James, G. (1963). Poverty as an obstacle to health progress in our cities. *American Journal of Public Health*, 55(11), 1758-1762.

62. Johnson, Spencer. (1985). *One Minute for Myself*. New York: Avon Books.

63. Johnston, D. W., Cook, D. G., and Shaper, A. G. (1987). Type A behaviour and ischaemic heart disease in middle-aged British men. *British Medical Journal*, 295: 86-89.

64. Kearns, Joseph L. (1973). *Stress in Industry*. London: Priory Press.

65. Kemple, C. (1945). Rorschach method and psychosomatic diagnosis. *Psychosomatic Medicine*, 7: 85-89.

66. Kobasa, Suzanne. (1982). The hardy personality: Toward a social psychology of stress and health. In J. Suls and G. Sanders (Eds.), *Social Psychology and Illness*. Hillsdale, NJ: Erlbaum.

67. Kornitzer, M., Kittel, F., DeBaker, G., and Dramaix, M. (1981). The Belgian Heart Disease Prevention Project: Type A behaviour pattern and the prevalence of coronary heart disease. *Psychosomatic Medicine*, 43: 313-320.

68. Le Masters, E. E. (1975). *Blue-Collar Aristocrats: Life-Styles at a Working Class Tavern*. Madison: University of Wisconsin Press.

69. Leshan, Lawrence. (1959). Psychological states as factors in the development of malignant disease: A critical review. *National Cancer Institute Journal*, 22: 1-18.

70. Leshan, Lawrence. (1975). *How to Meditate*. New York: Bantam Books.

71. Levi, Lennart. (1981). *Preventing Work Stress*. New York: Addison-Wesley.

72. Liddel, H. (1950). Some specific factors that modify tolerance for environmental stress. In H. G. Wolff, S. G. Wolff, and C. C. Hare (Eds.), *Life Stress and Bodily Disease*. Baltimore: Williams & Wilkins.

73. Likert, R. (1961). *New Patterns of Management*. New York: McGraw-Hill.

74. Lundberg, U., and Theonell, T. (1976). Scaling of life changes. Differences between three diagnostic groups and between recently experienced and non-experienced events. *Journal of Human Stress*, 2: 7-17.

75. Luthe, W. (1963). Autogenic training: Method, research and application in medicine. *American Journal of Psychotherapy*, 17: 174-195.

76. McKay, Matthew, and Fanning, Patrick. (1987). *Self-Esteem*. Oakland, CA: New Harbinger Publications.

77. McLean, Alan A. (Ed.) (1981). *Work Stress*. New York: Addison-Wesley.

78. Marmot, M. G., Rose, G., Shipley, M., and Hamilton, P. J. S. (1978). Employment grade and coronary heart disease in British civil servants. *Journal of Epidemiology and Community Health*, 32: 244-249.

79. Marmot, M. G., Syme, S. L., Kagan, A., Cohen, J. B., and Belsky, J. (1975). Epidemiologic studies of coronary heart disease and stroke in Japanese

men living in Japan, Hawaii and California: Prevalence of coronary and hypertensive heart disease and associated risk factors. *American Journal of Epidemiology*, 102(6): 514-525.

80. Marshall, Megan. (1984). *The Cost of Loving: Women and the New Fear of Intimacy.* New York: G. B. Putman.

81. Matsumoto, Y. S. (1970). Social stress and coronary heart disease in Japan: A hypothesis. *Millbank Memorial Fund Quarterly*, 48: 9-31.

82. Matthews, K. A., Glass, D. C., Rosenman, R. H., and Bortner, R. W. (1977). Competitive drive, pattern A and coronary heart disease: A further analysis of some data from the Western Collaborative Group Study. *Journal of Chronic Diseases*, 30: 489-498.

83. Matthews, Karen A. (1985). Assessment of type A behaviour, anger and hostility in epidemiological studies of cardiovasculur diseases. In A. M. Ostfeld and E.D. Eaker (Eds.), *Measuring Psychosocial Variables in Epidemiologic Studies of Cardiovascular Disease.* Proceedings of the NHLBI workshop NIH Publication No. 85-2270, Washington, DC: U.S. Government Printing Office.

84. Matthews, K. A., and Siegel, J. M. (1982). The Type A behaviour pattern in children and adolescents: assessment, development and associated coronary risk. In A. Baum and J. E. Singer (Eds.), *Handbook of Psychology and Health*, Vol. 2. Hillsdale, NJ: Erlbaum.

85. Maxwell-Hudson, Clare. (1988). *The Complete Book of Massage.* London: Dorling Kindersley.

86. Medalie, J. H., and Goldbourt, U. (1976). Angina pectoris among 10,000 men: II. Psychological and other risk factors as evidenced by a multivariate analysis of five year incidence study. *American Journal of Medicine*, 60: 910-921.

87. Meichenbaum, Donald. (1985). *Stress Inoculation Training.* New York: Pergamon.

88. Meichenbaum, Donald, and Jaremko, M. (1983). *Stress Reducing and Prevention.* New York: Plenum Press.

89. Menninger, K. A., and Menninger, W. C. (1936). Psychoanalytic observations in cardiac disorders. *American Heart Journal*, 11: 10-21.

90. Meyer, R. J., and Haggarty, R. J. (1962). Streptococcal infections in families. *Paediatrics*, 29: 539-549.

91. Moos, R. H., and Solomon, G. H. (1965). Psychologic comparisons between women with rheumatoid arthritis and their nonarthritic sisters. *Psychosomatic Medicine*, 2: 150.

92. Morris, Desmond. (1978). *Manwatching.* Frogmore, St. Albans: Triad Panther Books.

93. Multiple Risk Factor Intervention Trial (MRFIT) Research Group. (1979). Risk factor changes and mortality results. *Journal of American Medical Association*, 248: 1465-1477.

94. Narem, R. M., Levesque, M. J., and Cornhill, J. F. (1980). Social environment as a factor in diet-induced atherosclerosis. *Science*, 208: 1475-1476.
95. Ogilvie, H. (1949). In praise of idleness. *British Medical Journal*, 1: 645-651.
95a. Ornish, D. M., Brown, S. E., Scherwitz, L. W., Billings, J. H., Armstrong, W. T., Ports, T. A., McLananhan, S. M., Kirkeeide, R. L., Brand, R. J., and Gould, K. L. (1990). Can lifestyle change reverse coronary heart disease? *Lancet*, 336: 129-133.
96. Ornstein, R., and Sobel, D. (1988). *The Healing Brain*. New York: Macmillan.
97. Osler, W. (1910). The Lumlein Lectures on angina pectoris. *Lancet*, 1: 839-844.
98. Parkes, C. M., Benjamin, B., and Fitzgerald, R. G. (1969). Broken heart: A statistical study of increased mortality among widowers. *British Medical Journal*, 1: 740-743.
99. Patel, C. (1973). Yoga and biofeedback in the management of hypertension. *Lancet*, 2: 1053-1055.
100. Patel, C. (1987). *Fighting Heart Disease*. London: Dorling Kindersley.
101. Patel, C., and Marmot, M. G. (1987). Stress management, blood pressure and quality of life. *Journal of Hypertension*, 5, Supplement 1: 21-26.
102. Patel, Chandra, and Marmot, M. G. (1988). Can general practitioners use training in relaxation and management of stress to reduce mild hypertension? *British Medical Journal*, 296: 21-24.
103. Patel, Chandra, Marmot, M. G., Terry, D. J., Carruthers, M., Hunt, B., and Patel, M. (1985). Trial of relaxation in reducing coronary risk: Four year follow up. *British Medical Journal*, 290: 1103-1106.
104. Patel, Chandra, and North, W. R. S. (1975). Randomised controlled trial of yoga and biofeedback in the management of hypertension. *Lancet*, 2: 93-95.
105. Paykel, E. S. (1976). Life stress, depression and attempted suicide. *Journal of Human Stress*, 2: 3-12.
106. Pelletier, Kenneth. (Ed.) (1978). *Mind as Healer, Mind as Slayer*. London: George Allen & Unwin.
107. Pollak, C. P., Bradlow, H. G., Spielman, A. J., and Weitzman, E. D. (Eds.) (1979). A pilot survey of the symptoms of hypersomnia-sleep apnoea syndrome as possible prediction. *Sleep Research*, 8: 210.
108. Price, Virginia. (1982). *Type A Behaviour Pattern: A Model for Research and Practice*. New York: Academic Press.
109. Rahe, R. H. (1973). Life-change measurement as a predictor of illness. *Proceedings of the Royal Society of Medicine*, 61: 1124-1126.
110. Rama, Swami, Ballentine, Rudolph, and Hymes, Alan. (1979). *Science of Breath*. Honsdale, PA: Himalayan International Institute.

111. Raphael, B. (1977). Preventive intervention with the recently bereaved. *Archives of General Psychiatry*, 34: 1450-1454.
112. Redding, W. C. (1972). *Communication within the Organization: An Interpretative Review of Theory and Research*. New York: Industrial Communication Council.
113. Riddle, Patricia K. (1982). Chronic fatigue and women: A description and suggested treatment. *Women and Health*, 7(1): 37-38.
114. Rosenman, R. H., Brand, R. J., Jenkins, D., Friedman, M., Straus, R., and Wurm, M. (1975). Coronary heart disease in the Western Collaborative Group Study: Final follow-up experience of 8½ years. *Journal of the American Medical Association*, 233: 872-877.
115. Roskies, Ethel. (1987). *Stress Management for Health Type A*. New York: Guildford Press.
116. Russek, H. I. (1962). Emotional stress and coronary heart disease in American physicians, dentists and lawyers. *American Journal of Medical Science*, 243: 716-721.
117. Russek, H. I., and Zohman, R. L. (1958). Relative significance of heredity, diet and occupational stress in coronary heart disease of young adults. *American Journal of Medical Science*, 235: 266-277.
118. Schaef, Anne Wilson, and Fassel, Diane. (1988). Hooked on work. *New Age Journal*, January/February: 42. Farmingdale, NY.
119. Scherwitz, L., McKelvain, R., Laman, C., Patterson, J., Dutton, L., Yusim, S., Lester, J., Kraft, I., Rochelle, D., and Leachman, R. (1983). Type A behaviour, self-involvement, and coronary atherosclerosis. *Psychosomatic Medicine*, 45: 47-58.
120. Seligman, Martin E. P. (1975). *Helplessness*. San Francisco: W. H. Freeman.
121. Selye, Hans. (1975a). *Stress without Distress*. New York: Signet.
122. Selye, Hans. (1975b). *The Stress of Life*. New York: McGraw-Hill.
123. Shealy, C. Norman. (1977). *Ninety Days of Self-Health*. New York: Bantam Books.
124. Shekelle, R. B., Gayle, M., Ostfeld, A. M., and Paul, O. (1983). Hostility, risk of coronary heart disease and mortality. *Psychosomatic Medicine*, 45: 109-114.
125. Shostak, Arthur B. (1981). *Blue Collar Stress*. New York: Addison-Wesley.
126. Silva, Jose, with Miele, Philip. (1980). *The Silva Mind Control Method*. London: Grafton Books.
127. Simonton, Carl, Matthews-Simonton, Stephanie, and Creighton, James L. (1978). *Getting Well Again*. New York: Bantam Books.
128. Smedes, Lewis B. (1986). *Forget and Forgive*. New York: Pocket Books.
129. Smith, Manuel J. (1975). *When I Say No, I Feel Guilty*. New York: Bantam Books.

130. Sosa, Roberto, Kennel, J., and Klaus, M. (1980). The effect of a support-ive companion on parental problems, length of labor, and mother-infant interaction. *New England Journal of Medicine*, 303: 597-600.
131. Sroufe, Alan L. (1978). Attachment and the roots of competence. *Human Nature*, 1(10): 50-57.
132. Stout, G., Morrow, J., Brandt, E., and Wolf, S. (1964). Unusually low incidence of death from myocardial infarction in an Italian-American community in Pennsylvania. *Journal of American Medical Association*, 188: 845-849.
133. Tavris, Carol. (1982). *Anger: The Misunderstood Emotion*. New York: Simon & Schuster.
134. Thelle, D. S., Arnesen, E., and Forde, O. H. (1983). The Tromso Heart Study. *New England Journal of Medicine*, 308: 1454-1457.
135. Theoell, T. (1976). Selected illnesses and somatic factors in relation to two psychosocial stress indices—A prospective study of middle-aged con-struction building workers. *Journal of Psychosomatic Research*, 20: 7-20.
136. Theoell, T. (1985). Relationship between critical life events, job stress and cardiovascular illness. In D. W. Gentry, H. Benson, and C. J. de Wolff, *Behavioural Medicine: Work, Stress and Health*. Dordrecht: NATO ASI Series, Martinus Nijhoff Publishers.
137. Thomas, C. B., and Duszynski, K. R. (1974). Closeness to parents and the family constellation in a prospective study of five disease states: Suicide, mental illness, malignant tumour, hypertension and coronary heart disease. *The John Hopkins Medical Journal*, 134(5): 251-270.
138. Troxter, R. G., and Schwertner, H. A. (1985). Cholesterol, stress, life-style and coronary heart disease. *Aviation, Space and Environmental Medi-cine*, July, 660-665.
139. Veninga, R. L., and Spradley, J. (1981). *The Work/Stress Connection: How to Cope with Job Burnout*. Boston: Little, Brown.
140. Wallace, R. K., and Benson, H. (1972). The physiology of meditation. *Scientific American*, 226(2): 84-90.
141. Weiner, M. A. (1986). *Maximum Immunity*. Boston: Houghton Mifflin.
142. Willius, F. A., and Keys, T. A. (1941). *Cardiac Classics*. St. Louis, C. V. Mosby.
143. Wolf, S. G. (1958). Cardiovascular reactions to symbolic stimuli. *Circu-lation*, 18: 287-292.
144. Wolff, H. G. (1953). Changes in vulnerability of tissues: An aspect of man's response to threat. *The National Institute of Health Annual Lec-tures*. U.S. Department of Health, Education and Welfare Publication No. 388, 38-71.
145. Wolff, Harold G. (1963). *Headache and Other Head Pain*. Oxford: Ox-ford University Press.

146. Women's improved role: A mixed blessing? (1987). *The Watchtower*, August 15, London.
147. Work in America (1973). *Report of a Special Task Force to the Secretary of Health, Education and Welfare*. Cambridge: MIT Press.

Index